IBD Food Journal

INFORMATION

NAME

ADDRESS

E-MAIL ADDRESS

WEBSITE

PHONE   **FAX**

EMERGENCY CONTACT PERSON

PHONE   **FAX**

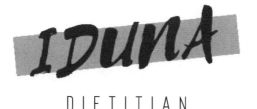

DIETITIAN

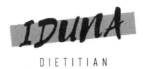

DIETITIAN

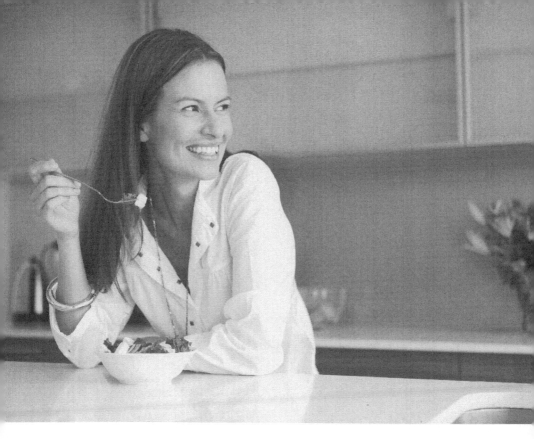

INTRODUCTION

Why diet in IBD is so important?

This disease affects the gastrointestinal tract, causing the formation of inflammatory changes in the affected focal sections. **These changes make the intestinal surface less able to absorb nutrients, vitamins, and minerals.**

The body does not get enough of what it needs for building and overall proper functioning, leading to **deficiencies**. As the disease progresses, the consequence may be the destruction of the organism.

Appropriate dietary and nutritional treatment, together with appropriate pharmacotherapy, **can delay or stop the development of the disease, keeping it in remission**.

Thanks to this, the person affected by this disease can lead a normal life. Studies show that people who follow the recommendations of doctors and nutritionists and do not give up nutritional therapy **achieve disease remission in 85%!**

General nutritional recommendations for IBD patients.

unfortunately, there is no ready-made nutrition system for a person with IBD. Each case should be dealt with individually.

The diet should not be radically different from that of healthy people, it should be balanced and adjusted to the age and weight of the patient. The patient should adhere to the following recommendations.

1. A patient should eat 4–5 small meals a day. Food consumed in this way is better tolerated and does not cause additional ailments in the patient.

2. The patient should eat easily digestible, therefore any bloating, spicy, or fried foods should be completely limited. He should also be careful about the drinks consumed, as drinking strong coffee and tea can aggravate the symptoms.

Difficult to digest foods may increase the number of bowel movements and aggravate pain in the abdominal cavity. Food products that can cause ailments include: **milk and its products, eggs, wheat, yeast, tomatoes, bananas, corn, and wine.**

3. Inflammation, fever, and increased cellular catabolism increase the patient's need for energy, which is why the patient is recommended an energy-rich diet. **Energy demand should be covered in 100-150%.**

4. The diet should be rich in protein (**tofu, lean meat, fish** is recommended) especially for people suffering from malnutrition as a result of illness.

5. Often, as a result of changes in the ileum, there is a reduction in the production of lactase (an enzyme that breaks down milk sugar - lactose), which is associated with poor tolerance of milk and its products. It manifests itself as diarrhea which can weaken the body. The consumption of milk is then limited. Fermented dairy products are usually better tolerated because they contain less lactose, but there are cases where they are also not tolerated. Then, lactase preparations can be administered as a dietary supplement.

Low consumption of dairy products and milk in people with low lactose tolerance may result in a deficiency of calcium and vitamin D, of which these foods are the main source. For this purpose, supplementation of these substances is necessary.

6. Vitamin supplementation from the group is recommended. **B, especially folic acid and vitamin B12** (deficiency causes macrocytic anemia), especially in people whose disease is located in the ileum, or as a result of its action, a significant part of the intestine has been removed.

7. Among the minerals, an adequate supply of **zinc** is important, as it strengthens the immune system, and its deficiency may, among other things, intensify diarrhea. Foods rich in zinc are **meat, offal, and oysters**, but if we are not able to cover the needs with a diet (because the condition of the sick person does not allow it), it is necessary to introduce supplementation.

8. The diet should be low in fat. Fat should account for only **20%** of the total energy of a food.

9. Omega-3 acids (mainly EPA, contained in fish oils) also positively affect the patient's condition, there are indications that the use of these acids supports remission, but there are no clear recommendations for their use.

10. More and more often we hear about the beneficial effects of **prebiotics**, reducing the level of pro-inflammatory cytokines in IBD disease, but research on this subject is still ongoing.

11. The patient should take care of the proper grinding of the consumed food by chewing it thoroughly.

12. The patient should consume a sufficient amount of fluids, as this prevents problems related to the passage of the digestive content.

Remember that these are general recommendations only.

Each organism reacts differently to different foods, which is why it is so **important to keep this journal diligently and observe the reactions to different foods.**

Concentrate more on the ingredients of your meals rather than your whole meals.

During the work of a dietitian, I encountered situations when the patient gave up all meals, and as it turned out later, the problem was an addition to this meal.

It is worth listing the ingredients of the meal. Later, it will be easier for you to determine which product is causing unpleasant consequences for you.

In IBD, it is also important to avoid tobacco, alcohol, and excessive stress.

Exercise and getting enough sleep can help.

It is also worth taking a moment every day to notice what we have achieved and personal reflections.

Follow all instructions and let that shit go!

DATE .... **WEIGHT** ....

BREAKFAST

....
....
....

TIME ....

PAIN LEVEL ① ② ③ ④ ⑤ ⑥ ⑦ ⑧ ⑨ ⑩

SYMPTOMS

☐ BLOODY STOOLS   ☐ DIARRHEA

☐ ABDOMINAL PAIN   ☐ FATIGUE

☐ REDUCED APPETITE   ☐ WEIGHT LOSS

☐ ....   ☐ ....

LUNCH

....
....
....

TIME ....

PAIN LEVEL ① ② ③ ④ ⑤ ⑥ ⑦ ⑧ ⑨ ⑩

SYMPTOMS

☐ BLOODY STOOLS   ☐ DIARRHEA

☐ ABDOMINAL PAIN   ☐ FATIGUE

☐ REDUCED APPETITE   ☐ WEIGHT LOSS

☐ ....   ☐ ....

DINNER

....
....
....

TIME ....

PAIN LEVEL ① ② ③ ④ ⑤ ⑥ ⑦ ⑧ ⑨ ⑩

SYMPTOMS

☐ BLOODY STOOLS   ☐ DIARRHEA

☐ ABDOMINAL PAIN   ☐ FATIGUE

☐ REDUCED APPETITE   ☐ WEIGHT LOSS

☐ ....   ☐ ....

SNACKS

....
....
....

TIME ....

PAIN LEVEL ① ② ③ ④ ⑤ ⑥ ⑦ ⑧ ⑨ ⑩

SYMPTOMS

☐ BLOODY STOOLS   ☐ DIARRHEA

☐ ABDOMINAL PAIN   ☐ FATIGUE

☐ REDUCED APPETITE   ☐ WEIGHT LOSS

☐ ....   ☐ ....

SNACKS

....
....
....

TIME ....

PAIN LEVEL ① ② ③ ④ ⑤ ⑥ ⑦ ⑧ ⑨ ⑩

SYMPTOMS

☐ BLOODY STOOLS   ☐ DIARRHEA

☐ ABDOMINAL PAIN   ☐ FATIGUE

☐ REDUCED APPETITE   ☐ WEIGHT LOSS

☐ ....   ☐ ....

MEDICATIONS & SUPPLEMENTS

....
....
....
....
....
....
....

EXTRA NOTES

....
....
....
....
....
....
....

Hours of Sleep

1	2	3	4	5
6	7	8	9	10

Physical Activity

....

....

....

Todays Mood

AVERAGE

POOR

GOOD

3

4

2

BAD

5

1

HAPPY

Energy Level

☐ ☐ ☐ ☐ ☐

Water Intake

Other Care Taken Today:

....

....

....

....

Bowel Movements

BM #1 ....   BM #2 ....   BM #3 ....   BM #4 ....

BM #5 ....   BM #6 ....   BM #7 ....   BM #8 ....

BM #9 ....   BM #10 ....   BM #11 ....   BM #12 ....

Todays Goals / Reflections

....

....

....

....

....

....

DATE _____   **WEIGHT** _____

BREAKFAST

....
....
....
....

TIME _____

PAIN LEVEL ① ② ③ ④ ⑤ ⑥ ⑦ ⑧ ⑨ ⑩

SYMPTOMS

☐ BLOODY STOOLS ☐ DIARRHEA
☐ ABDOMINAL PAIN ☐ FATIGUE
☐ REDUCED APPETITE ☐ WEIGHT LOSS
☐ .... ☐ ....

LUNCH

....
....
....
....

TIME _____

PAIN LEVEL ① ② ③ ④ ⑤ ⑥ ⑦ ⑧ ⑨ ⑩

SYMPTOMS

☐ BLOODY STOOLS ☐ DIARRHEA
☐ ABDOMINAL PAIN ☐ FATIGUE
☐ REDUCED APPETITE ☐ WEIGHT LOSS
☐ .... ☐ ....

DINNER

....
....
....
....

TIME _____

PAIN LEVEL ① ② ③ ④ ⑤ ⑥ ⑦ ⑧ ⑨ ⑩

SYMPTOMS

☐ BLOODY STOOLS ☐ DIARRHEA
☐ ABDOMINAL PAIN ☐ FATIGUE
☐ REDUCED APPETITE ☐ WEIGHT LOSS
☐ .... ☐ ....

SNACKS

....
....
....
....

TIME _____

PAIN LEVEL ① ② ③ ④ ⑤ ⑥ ⑦ ⑧ ⑨ ⑩

SYMPTOMS

☐ BLOODY STOOLS ☐ DIARRHEA
☐ ABDOMINAL PAIN ☐ FATIGUE
☐ REDUCED APPETITE ☐ WEIGHT LOSS
☐ .... ☐ ....

SNACKS

....
....
....
....

TIME _____

PAIN LEVEL ① ② ③ ④ ⑤ ⑥ ⑦ ⑧ ⑨ ⑩

SYMPTOMS

☐ BLOODY STOOLS ☐ DIARRHEA
☐ ABDOMINAL PAIN ☐ FATIGUE
☐ REDUCED APPETITE ☐ WEIGHT LOSS
☐ .... ☐ ....

MEDICATIONS & SUPPLEMENTS

....
....
....
....
....
....
....
....
....

EXTRA NOTES

....
....
....
....
....
....
....
....
....

Hours of Sleep

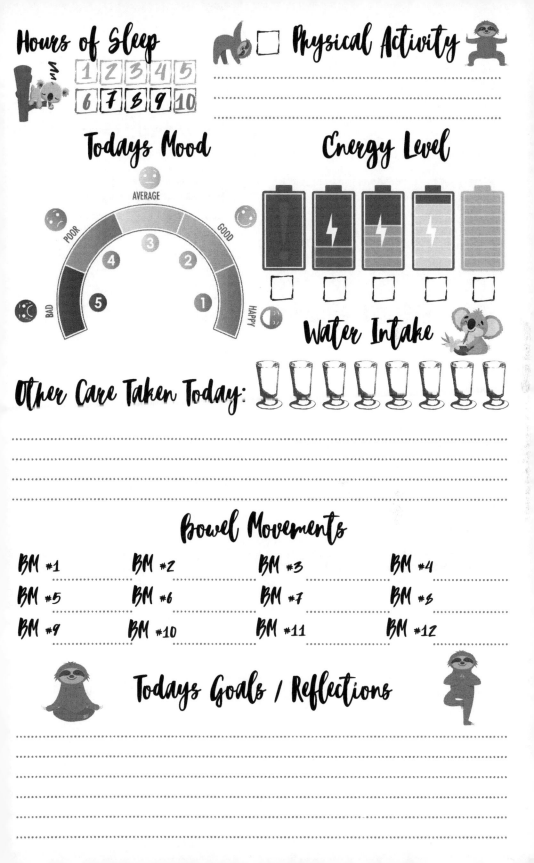

| 1 | 2 | 3 | 4 | 5 |
| 6 | 7 | 8 | 9 | 10 |

Physical Activity

☐

....
....
....

Todays Mood

AVERAGE
POOR
GOOD
4
3
2
5
1
BAD
HAPPY

Energy Level

☐ ☐ ☐ ☐ ☐

Water Intake

Other Care Taken Today:

....
....
....
....

Bowel Movements

BM #1 .... BM #2 .... BM #3 .... BM #4 ....

BM #5 .... BM #6 .... BM #7 .... BM #8 ....

BM #9 .... BM #10 .... BM #11 .... BM #12 ....

Todays Goals / Reflections

....
....
....
....
....
....

DATE _____ **WEIGHT** _____

BREAKFAST

....
....
....
....

TIME _____

PAIN LEVEL ① ② ③ ④ ⑤ ⑥ ⑦ ⑧ ⑨ ⑩

SYMPTOMS

☐ BLOODY STOOLS   ☐ DIARRHEA
☐ ABDOMINAL PAIN   ☐ FATIGUE
☐ REDUCED APPETITE   ☐ WEIGHT LOSS
☐ ....   ☐ ....

LUNCH

....
....
....
....

TIME _____

PAIN LEVEL ① ② ③ ④ ⑤ ⑥ ⑦ ⑧ ⑨ ⑩

SYMPTOMS

☐ BLOODY STOOLS   ☐ DIARRHEA
☐ ABDOMINAL PAIN   ☐ FATIGUE
☐ REDUCED APPETITE   ☐ WEIGHT LOSS
☐ ....   ☐ ....

DINNER

....
....
....
....

TIME _____

PAIN LEVEL ① ② ③ ④ ⑤ ⑥ ⑦ ⑧ ⑨ ⑩

SYMPTOMS

☐ BLOODY STOOLS   ☐ DIARRHEA
☐ ABDOMINAL PAIN   ☐ FATIGUE
☐ REDUCED APPETITE   ☐ WEIGHT LOSS
☐ ....   ☐ ....

SNACKS

....
....
....
....

TIME _____

PAIN LEVEL ① ② ③ ④ ⑤ ⑥ ⑦ ⑧ ⑨ ⑩

SYMPTOMS

☐ BLOODY STOOLS   ☐ DIARRHEA
☐ ABDOMINAL PAIN   ☐ FATIGUE
☐ REDUCED APPETITE   ☐ WEIGHT LOSS
☐ ....   ☐ ....

SNACKS

....
....
....
....

TIME _____

PAIN LEVEL ① ② ③ ④ ⑤ ⑥ ⑦ ⑧ ⑨ ⑩

SYMPTOMS

☐ BLOODY STOOLS   ☐ DIARRHEA
☐ ABDOMINAL PAIN   ☐ FATIGUE
☐ REDUCED APPETITE   ☐ WEIGHT LOSS
☐ ....   ☐ ....

MEDICATIONS & SUPPLEMENTS

....
....
....
....
....
....
....
....
....

EXTRA NOTES

....
....
....
....
....
....
....
....
....

Hours of Sleep

| 1 | 2 | 3 | 4 | 5 |
| 6 | 7 | 8 | 9 | 10 |

☐ Physical Activity

....
....

Todays Mood

AVERAGE
POOR
GOOD
BAD
HAPPY

3
4
2
5
1

Energy Level

☐ ☐ ☐ ☐ ☐

Water Intake

Other Care Taken Today:

....
....
....
....

Bowel Movements

BM #1	BM #2	BM #3	BM #4
BM #5	BM #6	BM #7	BM #8
BM #9	BM #10	BM #11	BM #12

Todays Goals / Reflections

....
....
....
....
....

DATE _____   **WEIGHT** _____

BREAKFAST

....
....
....
....

TIME _____

PAIN LEVEL (1)(2)(3)(4)(5)(6)(7)(8)(9)(10)

SYMPTOMS

☐ BLOODY STOOLS   ☐ DIARRHEA

☐ ABDOMINAL PAIN   ☐ FATIGUE

☐ REDUCED APPETITE ☐ WEIGHT LOSS

☐ .... ☐ ....

LUNCH

....
....
....
....

TIME _____

PAIN LEVEL (1)(2)(3)(4)(5)(6)(7)(8)(9)(10)

SYMPTOMS

☐ BLOODY STOOLS   ☐ DIARRHEA

☐ ABDOMINAL PAIN   ☐ FATIGUE

☐ REDUCED APPETITE ☐ WEIGHT LOSS

☐ .... ☐ ....

DINNER

....
....
....
....

TIME _____

PAIN LEVEL (1)(2)(3)(4)(5)(6)(7)(8)(9)(10)

SYMPTOMS

☐ BLOODY STOOLS   ☐ DIARRHEA

☐ ABDOMINAL PAIN   ☐ FATIGUE

☐ REDUCED APPETITE ☐ WEIGHT LOSS

☐ .... ☐ ....

SNACKS

....
....
....
....

TIME _____

PAIN LEVEL (1)(2)(3)(4)(5)(6)(7)(8)(9)(10)

SYMPTOMS

☐ BLOODY STOOLS   ☐ DIARRHEA

☐ ABDOMINAL PAIN   ☐ FATIGUE

☐ REDUCED APPETITE ☐ WEIGHT LOSS

☐ .... ☐ ....

SNACKS

....
....
....
....

TIME _____

PAIN LEVEL (1)(2)(3)(4)(5)(6)(7)(8)(9)(10)

SYMPTOMS

☐ BLOODY STOOLS   ☐ DIARRHEA

☐ ABDOMINAL PAIN   ☐ FATIGUE

☐ REDUCED APPETITE ☐ WEIGHT LOSS

☐ .... ☐ ....

MEDICATIONS & SUPPLEMENTS

....
....
....
....
....
....
....
....
....
....

EXTRA NOTES

....
....
....
....
....
....
....
....
....
....

Hours of Sleep

| 1 | 2 | 3 | 4 | 5 |
| 6 | 7 | 8 | 9 | 10 |

Physical Activity

....

....

....

Todays Mood

POOR

AVERAGE

GOOD

BAD

HAPPY

3

4

2

5

1

Energy Level

☐ ☐ ☐ ☐ ☐

Water Intake

Other Care Taken Today:

....

....

....

....

Bowel Movements

BM #1 .... BM #2 .... BM #3 .... BM #4 ....

BM #5 .... BM #6 .... BM #7 .... BM #8 ....

BM #9 .... BM #10 .... BM #11 .... BM #12 ....

Todays Goals / Reflections

....

....

....

....

....

DATE _____ **WEIGHT** _____

BREAKFAST

....
....
....
....

TIME _____

PAIN LEVEL ① ② ③ ④ ⑤ ⑥ ⑦ ⑧ ⑨ ⑩

SYMPTOMS

☐ BLOODY STOOLS   ☐ DIARRHEA

☐ ABDOMINAL PAIN   ☐ FATIGUE

☐ REDUCED APPETITE   ☐ WEIGHT LOSS

☐ ....   ☐ ....

LUNCH

....
....
....
....

TIME _____

PAIN LEVEL ① ② ③ ④ ⑤ ⑥ ⑦ ⑧ ⑨ ⑩

SYMPTOMS

☐ BLOODY STOOLS   ☐ DIARRHEA

☐ ABDOMINAL PAIN   ☐ FATIGUE

☐ REDUCED APPETITE   ☐ WEIGHT LOSS

☐ ....   ☐ ....

DINNER

....
....
....
....

TIME _____

PAIN LEVEL ① ② ③ ④ ⑤ ⑥ ⑦ ⑧ ⑨ ⑩

SYMPTOMS

☐ BLOODY STOOLS   ☐ DIARRHEA

☐ ABDOMINAL PAIN   ☐ FATIGUE

☐ REDUCED APPETITE   ☐ WEIGHT LOSS

☐ ....   ☐ ....

SNACKS

....
....
....
....

TIME _____

PAIN LEVEL ① ② ③ ④ ⑤ ⑥ ⑦ ⑧ ⑨ ⑩

SYMPTOMS

☐ BLOODY STOOLS   ☐ DIARRHEA

☐ ABDOMINAL PAIN   ☐ FATIGUE

☐ REDUCED APPETITE   ☐ WEIGHT LOSS

☐ ....   ☐ ....

SNACKS

....
....
....
....

TIME _____

PAIN LEVEL ① ② ③ ④ ⑤ ⑥ ⑦ ⑧ ⑨ ⑩

SYMPTOMS

☐ BLOODY STOOLS   ☐ DIARRHEA

☐ ABDOMINAL PAIN   ☐ FATIGUE

☐ REDUCED APPETITE   ☐ WEIGHT LOSS

☐ ....   ☐ ....

MEDICATIONS & SUPPLEMENTS

....
....
....
....
....
....
....
....

EXTRA NOTES

....
....
....
....
....
....
....
....

Hours of Sleep

| 1 | 2 | 3 | 4 | 5 |
| 6 | 7 | 8 | 9 | 10 |

Physical Activity

☐

....
....
....

Todays Mood

POOR — AVERAGE — GOOD

3
4 · 2
5 · 1

BAD · HAPPY

Energy Level

☐ ☐ ☐ ☐ ☐

Water Intake

Other Care Taken Today:

....
....
....
....

Bowel Movements

BM #1	BM #2	BM #3	BM #4
BM #5	BM #6	BM #7	BM #8
BM #9	BM #10	BM #11	BM #12

Todays Goals / Reflections

....
....
....
....
....
....

DATE _____ **WEIGHT** _____

BREAKFAST

....
....
....
....

TIME _____

PAIN LEVEL ① ② ③ ④ ⑤ ⑥ ⑦ ⑧ ⑨ ⑩

SYMPTOMS

☐ BLOODY STOOLS ☐ DIARRHEA
☐ ABDOMINAL PAIN ☐ FATIGUE
☐ REDUCED APPETITE ☐ WEIGHT LOSS
☐ .... ☐ ....

LUNCH

....
....
....
....

TIME _____

PAIN LEVEL ① ② ③ ④ ⑤ ⑥ ⑦ ⑧ ⑨ ⑩

SYMPTOMS

☐ BLOODY STOOLS ☐ DIARRHEA
☐ ABDOMINAL PAIN ☐ FATIGUE
☐ REDUCED APPETITE ☐ WEIGHT LOSS
☐ .... ☐ ....

DINNER

....
....
....
....

TIME _____

PAIN LEVEL ① ② ③ ④ ⑤ ⑥ ⑦ ⑧ ⑨ ⑩

SYMPTOMS

☐ BLOODY STOOLS ☐ DIARRHEA
☐ ABDOMINAL PAIN ☐ FATIGUE
☐ REDUCED APPETITE ☐ WEIGHT LOSS
☐ .... ☐ ....

SNACKS

....
....
....
....

TIME _____

PAIN LEVEL ① ② ③ ④ ⑤ ⑥ ⑦ ⑧ ⑨ ⑩

SYMPTOMS

☐ BLOODY STOOLS ☐ DIARRHEA
☐ ABDOMINAL PAIN ☐ FATIGUE
☐ REDUCED APPETITE ☐ WEIGHT LOSS
☐ .... ☐ ....

SNACKS

....
....
....
....

TIME _____

PAIN LEVEL ① ② ③ ④ ⑤ ⑥ ⑦ ⑧ ⑨ ⑩

SYMPTOMS

☐ BLOODY STOOLS ☐ DIARRHEA
☐ ABDOMINAL PAIN ☐ FATIGUE
☐ REDUCED APPETITE ☐ WEIGHT LOSS
☐ .... ☐ ....

MEDICATIONS & SUPPLEMENTS

....
....
....
....
....
....
....
....
....
....

EXTRA NOTES

....
....
....
....
....
....
....
....
....
....

Hours of Sleep

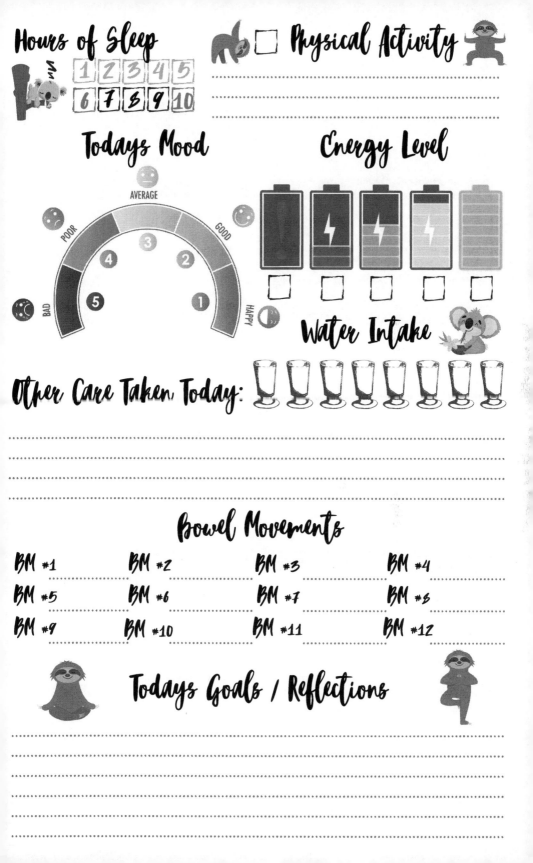

1	2	3	4	5
6	7	8	9	10

Physical Activity

....
....
....

Todays Mood

POOR
AVERAGE
GOOD
BAD
HAPPY

3
4
2
5
1

Energy Level

☐ ☐ ☐ ☐ ☐

Water Intake

Other Care Taken Today:

....
....
....
....

Bowel Movements

BM #1	BM #2	BM #3	BM #4
BM #5	BM #6	BM #7	BM #8
BM #9	BM #10	BM #11	BM #12

Todays Goals / Reflections

....
....
....
....
....
....

DATE _____ **WEIGHT** _____

BREAKFAST

....
....
....
....

TIME _____

PAIN LEVEL ① ② ③ ④ ⑤ ⑥ ⑦ ⑧ ⑨ ⑩

SYMPTOMS

☐ BLOODY STOOLS   ☐ DIARRHEA
☐ ABDOMINAL PAIN ☐ FATIGUE
☐ REDUCED APPETITE ☐ WEIGHT LOSS
☐ .... ☐ ....

LUNCH

....
....
....
....

TIME _____

PAIN LEVEL ① ② ③ ④ ⑤ ⑥ ⑦ ⑧ ⑨ ⑩

SYMPTOMS

☐ BLOODY STOOLS   ☐ DIARRHEA
☐ ABDOMINAL PAIN ☐ FATIGUE
☐ REDUCED APPETITE ☐ WEIGHT LOSS
☐ .... ☐ ....

DINNER

....
....
....
....

TIME _____

PAIN LEVEL ① ② ③ ④ ⑤ ⑥ ⑦ ⑧ ⑨ ⑩

SYMPTOMS

☐ BLOODY STOOLS   ☐ DIARRHEA
☐ ABDOMINAL PAIN ☐ FATIGUE
☐ REDUCED APPETITE ☐ WEIGHT LOSS
☐ .... ☐ ....

SNACKS

....
....
....
....

TIME _____

PAIN LEVEL ① ② ③ ④ ⑤ ⑥ ⑦ ⑧ ⑨ ⑩

SYMPTOMS

☐ BLOODY STOOLS   ☐ DIARRHEA
☐ ABDOMINAL PAIN ☐ FATIGUE
☐ REDUCED APPETITE ☐ WEIGHT LOSS
☐ .... ☐ ....

SNACKS

....
....
....
....

TIME _____

PAIN LEVEL ① ② ③ ④ ⑤ ⑥ ⑦ ⑧ ⑨ ⑩

SYMPTOMS

☐ BLOODY STOOLS   ☐ DIARRHEA
☐ ABDOMINAL PAIN ☐ FATIGUE
☐ REDUCED APPETITE ☐ WEIGHT LOSS
☐ .... ☐ ....

MEDICATIONS & SUPPLEMENTS

....
....
....
....
....
....
....
....

EXTRA NOTES

....
....
....
....
....
....
....
....

Hours of Sleep

1	2	3	4	5
6	7	8	9	10

☐ Physical Activity

....
....
....

Todays Mood

AVERAGE

POOR

GOOD

3

4

2

BAD

5

1

HAPPY

Energy Level

☐ ☐ ☐ ☐ ☐

Water Intake

Other Care Taken Today:

....
....
....
....

Bowel Movements

BM #1	BM #2	BM #3	BM #4
BM #5	BM #6	BM #7	BM #8
BM #9	BM #10	BM #11	BM #12

Todays Goals / Reflections

....
....
....
....
....

DATE _____   **WEIGHT** _____

BREAKFAST

....
....
....
....

TIME _____

PAIN LEVEL ① ② ③ ④ ⑤ ⑥ ⑦ ⑧ ⑨ ⑩

SYMPTOMS

☐ BLOODY STOOLS   ☐ DIARRHEA
☐ ABDOMINAL PAIN   ☐ FATIGUE
☐ REDUCED APPETITE   ☐ WEIGHT LOSS
☐ ....   ☐ ....

LUNCH

....
....
....
....

TIME _____

PAIN LEVEL ① ② ③ ④ ⑤ ⑥ ⑦ ⑧ ⑨ ⑩

SYMPTOMS

☐ BLOODY STOOLS   ☐ DIARRHEA
☐ ABDOMINAL PAIN   ☐ FATIGUE
☐ REDUCED APPETITE   ☐ WEIGHT LOSS
☐ ....   ☐ ....

DINNER

....
....
....
....

TIME _____

PAIN LEVEL ① ② ③ ④ ⑤ ⑥ ⑦ ⑧ ⑨ ⑩

SYMPTOMS

☐ BLOODY STOOLS   ☐ DIARRHEA
☐ ABDOMINAL PAIN   ☐ FATIGUE
☐ REDUCED APPETITE   ☐ WEIGHT LOSS
☐ ....   ☐ ....

SNACKS

....
....
....
....

TIME _____

PAIN LEVEL ① ② ③ ④ ⑤ ⑥ ⑦ ⑧ ⑨ ⑩

SYMPTOMS

☐ BLOODY STOOLS   ☐ DIARRHEA
☐ ABDOMINAL PAIN   ☐ FATIGUE
☐ REDUCED APPETITE   ☐ WEIGHT LOSS
☐ ....   ☐ ....

SNACKS

....
....
....
....

TIME _____

PAIN LEVEL ① ② ③ ④ ⑤ ⑥ ⑦ ⑧ ⑨ ⑩

SYMPTOMS

☐ BLOODY STOOLS   ☐ DIARRHEA
☐ ABDOMINAL PAIN   ☐ FATIGUE
☐ REDUCED APPETITE   ☐ WEIGHT LOSS
☐ ....   ☐ ....

MEDICATIONS & SUPPLEMENTS

....
....
....
....
....
....
....
....
....
....

EXTRA NOTES

....
....
....
....
....
....
....
....
....
....

Hours of Sleep

1	2	3	4	5
6	7	8	9	10

Physical Activity

☐

....
....
....

Todays Mood

AVERAGE
POOR
GOOD
3
4
2
BAD
5
1
HAPPY

Energy Level

☐ ☐ ☐ ☐ ☐

Water Intake

Other Care Taken Today:

....
....
....
....

Bowel Movements

BM #1 ....

BM #2 ....

BM #3 ....

BM #4 ....

BM #5 ....

BM #6 ....

BM #7 ....

BM #8 ....

BM #9 ....

BM #10 ....

BM #11 ....

BM #12 ....

Todays Goals / Reflections

....
....
....
....
....
....

DATE _____ **WEIGHT** _____

BREAKFAST

....
....
....
....

TIME _____

PAIN LEVEL ① ② ③ ④ ⑤ ⑥ ⑦ ⑧ ⑨ ⑩

SYMPTOMS

☐ BLOODY STOOLS ☐ DIARRHEA

☐ ABDOMINAL PAIN ☐ FATIGUE

☐ REDUCED APPETITE ☐ WEIGHT LOSS

☐ .... ☐ ....

LUNCH

....
....
....
....

TIME _____

PAIN LEVEL ① ② ③ ④ ⑤ ⑥ ⑦ ⑧ ⑨ ⑩

SYMPTOMS

☐ BLOODY STOOLS ☐ DIARRHEA

☐ ABDOMINAL PAIN ☐ FATIGUE

☐ REDUCED APPETITE ☐ WEIGHT LOSS

☐ .... ☐ ....

DINNER

....
....
....
....

TIME _____

PAIN LEVEL ① ② ③ ④ ⑤ ⑥ ⑦ ⑧ ⑨ ⑩

SYMPTOMS

☐ BLOODY STOOLS ☐ DIARRHEA

☐ ABDOMINAL PAIN ☐ FATIGUE

☐ REDUCED APPETITE ☐ WEIGHT LOSS

☐ .... ☐ ....

SNACKS

....
....
....
....

TIME _____

PAIN LEVEL ① ② ③ ④ ⑤ ⑥ ⑦ ⑧ ⑨ ⑩

SYMPTOMS

☐ BLOODY STOOLS ☐ DIARRHEA

☐ ABDOMINAL PAIN ☐ FATIGUE

☐ REDUCED APPETITE ☐ WEIGHT LOSS

☐ .... ☐ ....

SNACKS

....
....
....
....

TIME _____

PAIN LEVEL ① ② ③ ④ ⑤ ⑥ ⑦ ⑧ ⑨ ⑩

SYMPTOMS

☐ BLOODY STOOLS ☐ DIARRHEA

☐ ABDOMINAL PAIN ☐ FATIGUE

☐ REDUCED APPETITE ☐ WEIGHT LOSS

☐ .... ☐ ....

MEDICATIONS & SUPPLEMENTS

....
....
....
....
....
....
....
....
....

EXTRA NOTES

....
....
....
....
....
....
....
....
....

Hours of Sleep

1	2	3	4	5
6	7	8	9	10

Physical Activity ☐

....

....

....

Todays Mood

AVERAGE

POOR

GOOD

3

4

2

5

1

BAD

HAPPY

Energy Level

☐ ☐ ☐ ☐ ☐

Water Intake

Other Care Taken Today:

....

....

....

....

Bowel Movements

BM #1	BM #2	BM #3	BM #4
BM #5	BM #6	BM #7	BM #8
BM #9	BM #10	BM #11	BM #12

Todays Goals / Reflections

....

....

....

....

....

....

DATE _____   **WEIGHT** _____

BREAKFAST

....
....
....
....

TIME _____

PAIN LEVEL (1) (2) (3) (4) (5) (6) (7) (8) (9) (10)

SYMPTOMS

☐ BLOODY STOOLS   ☐ DIARRHEA
☐ ABDOMINAL PAIN   ☐ FATIGUE
☐ REDUCED APPETITE   ☐ WEIGHT LOSS
☐ ....   ☐ ....

LUNCH

....
....
....
....

TIME _____

PAIN LEVEL (1) (2) (3) (4) (5) (6) (7) (8) (9) (10)

SYMPTOMS

☐ BLOODY STOOLS   ☐ DIARRHEA
☐ ABDOMINAL PAIN   ☐ FATIGUE
☐ REDUCED APPETITE   ☐ WEIGHT LOSS
☐ ....   ☐ ....

DINNER

....
....
....
....

TIME _____

PAIN LEVEL (1) (2) (3) (4) (5) (6) (7) (8) (9) (10)

SYMPTOMS

☐ BLOODY STOOLS   ☐ DIARRHEA
☐ ABDOMINAL PAIN   ☐ FATIGUE
☐ REDUCED APPETITE   ☐ WEIGHT LOSS
☐ ....   ☐ ....

SNACKS

....
....
....
....

TIME _____

PAIN LEVEL (1) (2) (3) (4) (5) (6) (7) (8) (9) (10)

SYMPTOMS

☐ BLOODY STOOLS   ☐ DIARRHEA
☐ ABDOMINAL PAIN   ☐ FATIGUE
☐ REDUCED APPETITE   ☐ WEIGHT LOSS
☐ ....   ☐ ....

SNACKS

....
....
....
....

TIME _____

PAIN LEVEL (1) (2) (3) (4) (5) (6) (7) (8) (9) (10)

SYMPTOMS

☐ BLOODY STOOLS   ☐ DIARRHEA
☐ ABDOMINAL PAIN   ☐ FATIGUE
☐ REDUCED APPETITE   ☐ WEIGHT LOSS
☐ ....   ☐ ....

MEDICATIONS & SUPPLEMENTS

....
....
....
....
....
....
....
....
....

EXTRA NOTES

....
....
....
....
....
....
....
....
....

Hours of Sleep

| 1 | 2 | 3 | 4 | 5 |
| 6 | 7 | 8 | 9 | 10 |

Physical Activity

☐

....
....
....

Todays Mood

AVERAGE

POOR

GOOD

3

4

2

5

1

BAD

HAPPY

Energy Level

☐ ☐ ☐ ☐ ☐

Water Intake

Other Care Taken Today:

....
....
....
....

Bowel Movements

BM #1 ....

BM #2 ....

BM #3 ....

BM #4 ....

BM #5 ....

BM #6 ....

BM #7 ....

BM #8 ....

BM #9 ....

BM #10 ....

BM #11 ....

BM #12 ....

Todays Goals / Reflections

....
....
....
....
....
....

DATE _____   WEIGHT _____

BREAKFAST

....
....
....
....

TIME _____

PAIN LEVEL ① ② ③ ④ ⑤ ⑥ ⑦ ⑧ ⑨ ⑩

SYMPTOMS

☐ BLOODY STOOLS   ☐ DIARRHEA
☐ ABDOMINAL PAIN   ☐ FATIGUE
☐ REDUCED APPETITE   ☐ WEIGHT LOSS
☐ .... ☐ ....

LUNCH

....
....
....
....

TIME _____

PAIN LEVEL ① ② ③ ④ ⑤ ⑥ ⑦ ⑧ ⑨ ⑩

SYMPTOMS

☐ BLOODY STOOLS   ☐ DIARRHEA
☐ ABDOMINAL PAIN   ☐ FATIGUE
☐ REDUCED APPETITE   ☐ WEIGHT LOSS
☐ .... ☐ ....

DINNER

....
....
....
....

TIME _____

PAIN LEVEL ① ② ③ ④ ⑤ ⑥ ⑦ ⑧ ⑨ ⑩

SYMPTOMS

☐ BLOODY STOOLS   ☐ DIARRHEA
☐ ABDOMINAL PAIN   ☐ FATIGUE
☐ REDUCED APPETITE   ☐ WEIGHT LOSS
☐ .... ☐ ....

SNACKS

....
....
....
....

TIME _____

PAIN LEVEL ① ② ③ ④ ⑤ ⑥ ⑦ ⑧ ⑨ ⑩

SYMPTOMS

☐ BLOODY STOOLS   ☐ DIARRHEA
☐ ABDOMINAL PAIN   ☐ FATIGUE
☐ REDUCED APPETITE   ☐ WEIGHT LOSS
☐ .... ☐ ....

SNACKS

....
....
....
....

TIME _____

PAIN LEVEL ① ② ③ ④ ⑤ ⑥ ⑦ ⑧ ⑨ ⑩

SYMPTOMS

☐ BLOODY STOOLS   ☐ DIARRHEA
☐ ABDOMINAL PAIN   ☐ FATIGUE
☐ REDUCED APPETITE   ☐ WEIGHT LOSS
☐ .... ☐ ....

MEDICATIONS & SUPPLEMENTS

....
....
....
....
....
....
....
....
....
....

EXTRA NOTES

....
....
....
....
....
....
....
....
....
....

Hours of Sleep

1	2	3	4	5
6	7	8	9	10

Physical Activity

....
....

Todays Mood

POOR
AVERAGE
GOOD
BAD
HAPPY

3
4
2
5
1

Energy Level

☐ ☐ ☐ ☐ ☐

Water Intake

Other Care Taken Today:

....
....
....
....

Bowel Movements

BM #1	BM #2	BM #3	BM #4
BM #5	BM #6	BM #7	BM #8
BM #9	BM #10	BM #11	BM #12

Todays Goals / Reflections

....
....
....
....
....
....

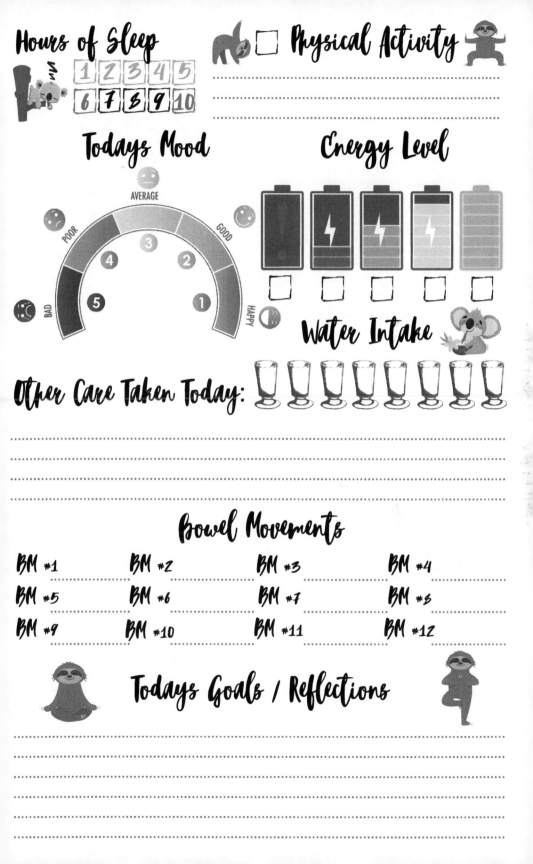

DATE _____ **WEIGHT** _____

BREAKFAST

....
....
....
....

TIME _____

PAIN LEVEL (1)(2)(3)(4)(5)(6)(7)(8)(9)(10)

SYMPTOMS

☐ BLOODY STOOLS   ☐ DIARRHEA
☐ ABDOMINAL PAIN   ☐ FATIGUE
☐ REDUCED APPETITE   ☐ WEIGHT LOSS
☐ .... ☐ ....

LUNCH

....
....
....
....

TIME _____

PAIN LEVEL (1)(2)(3)(4)(5)(6)(7)(8)(9)(10)

SYMPTOMS

☐ BLOODY STOOLS   ☐ DIARRHEA
☐ ABDOMINAL PAIN   ☐ FATIGUE
☐ REDUCED APPETITE   ☐ WEIGHT LOSS
☐ .... ☐ ....

DINNER

....
....
....
....

TIME _____

PAIN LEVEL (1)(2)(3)(4)(5)(6)(7)(8)(9)(10)

SYMPTOMS

☐ BLOODY STOOLS   ☐ DIARRHEA
☐ ABDOMINAL PAIN   ☐ FATIGUE
☐ REDUCED APPETITE   ☐ WEIGHT LOSS
☐ .... ☐ ....

SNACKS

....
....
....
....

TIME _____

PAIN LEVEL (1)(2)(3)(4)(5)(6)(7)(8)(9)(10)

SYMPTOMS

☐ BLOODY STOOLS   ☐ DIARRHEA
☐ ABDOMINAL PAIN   ☐ FATIGUE
☐ REDUCED APPETITE   ☐ WEIGHT LOSS
☐ .... ☐ ....

SNACKS

....
....
....
....

TIME _____

PAIN LEVEL (1)(2)(3)(4)(5)(6)(7)(8)(9)(10)

SYMPTOMS

☐ BLOODY STOOLS   ☐ DIARRHEA
☐ ABDOMINAL PAIN   ☐ FATIGUE
☐ REDUCED APPETITE   ☐ WEIGHT LOSS
☐ .... ☐ ....

MEDICATIONS & SUPPLEMENTS

....
....
....
....
....
....
....
....
....
....

EXTRA NOTES

....
....
....
....
....
....
....
....
....
....

Hours of Sleep

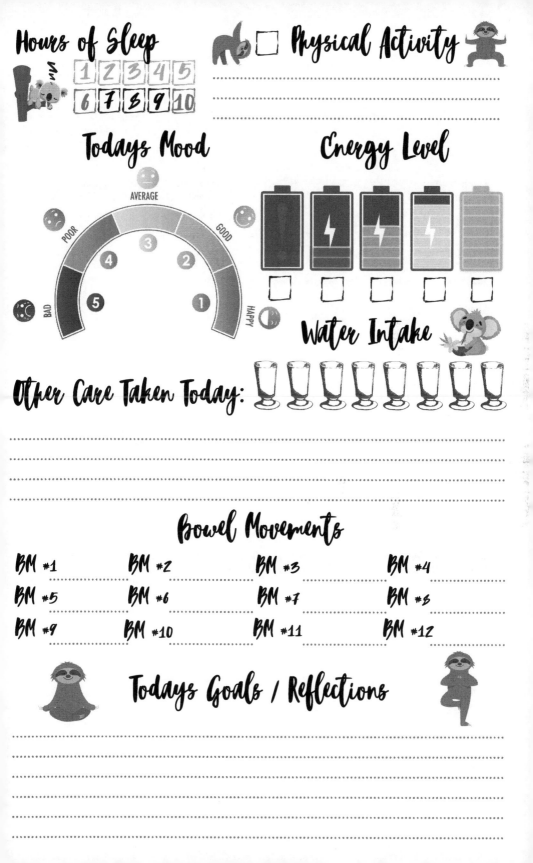

1	2	3	4	5
6	7	8	9	10

Physical Activity

....
....
....

Todays Mood

AVERAGE

POOR

GOOD

3

4

2

BAD

5

1

HAPPY

Energy Level

☐ ☐ ☐ ☐ ☐

Water Intake

Other Care Taken Today:

....
....
....
....

Bowel Movements

BM #1	BM #2	BM #3	BM #4
BM #5	BM #6	BM #7	BM #8
BM #9	BM #10	BM #11	BM #12

Todays Goals / Reflections

....
....
....
....
....
....

DATE　　　　　　　　　　　　　　　　**WEIGHT**

BREAKFAST

....
....
....
....

TIME

PAIN LEVEL　① ② ③ ④ ⑤ ⑥ ⑦ ⑧ ⑨ ⑩

SYMPTOMS

☐ BLOODY STOOLS　　☐ DIARRHEA

☐ ABDOMINAL PAIN　　☐ FATIGUE

☐ REDUCED APPETITE　☐ WEIGHT LOSS

☐ ....　☐ ....

LUNCH

....
....
....
....

TIME

PAIN LEVEL　① ② ③ ④ ⑤ ⑥ ⑦ ⑧ ⑨ ⑩

SYMPTOMS

☐ BLOODY STOOLS　　☐ DIARRHEA

☐ ABDOMINAL PAIN　　☐ FATIGUE

☐ REDUCED APPETITE　☐ WEIGHT LOSS

☐ ....　☐ ....

DINNER

....
....
....
....

TIME

PAIN LEVEL　① ② ③ ④ ⑤ ⑥ ⑦ ⑧ ⑨ ⑩

SYMPTOMS

☐ BLOODY STOOLS　　☐ DIARRHEA

☐ ABDOMINAL PAIN　　☐ FATIGUE

☐ REDUCED APPETITE　☐ WEIGHT LOSS

☐ ....　☐ ....

SNACKS

....
....
....
....

TIME

PAIN LEVEL　① ② ③ ④ ⑤ ⑥ ⑦ ⑧ ⑨ ⑩

SYMPTOMS

☐ BLOODY STOOLS　　☐ DIARRHEA

☐ ABDOMINAL PAIN　　☐ FATIGUE

☐ REDUCED APPETITE　☐ WEIGHT LOSS

☐ ....　☐ ....

SNACKS

....
....
....
....

TIME

PAIN LEVEL　① ② ③ ④ ⑤ ⑥ ⑦ ⑧ ⑨ ⑩

SYMPTOMS

☐ BLOODY STOOLS　　☐ DIARRHEA

☐ ABDOMINAL PAIN　　☐ FATIGUE

☐ REDUCED APPETITE　☐ WEIGHT LOSS

☐ ....　☐ ....

MEDICATIONS & SUPPLEMENTS

....
....
....
....
....
....
....
....
....
....

EXTRA NOTES

....
....
....
....
....
....
....
....
....
....

Hours of Sleep

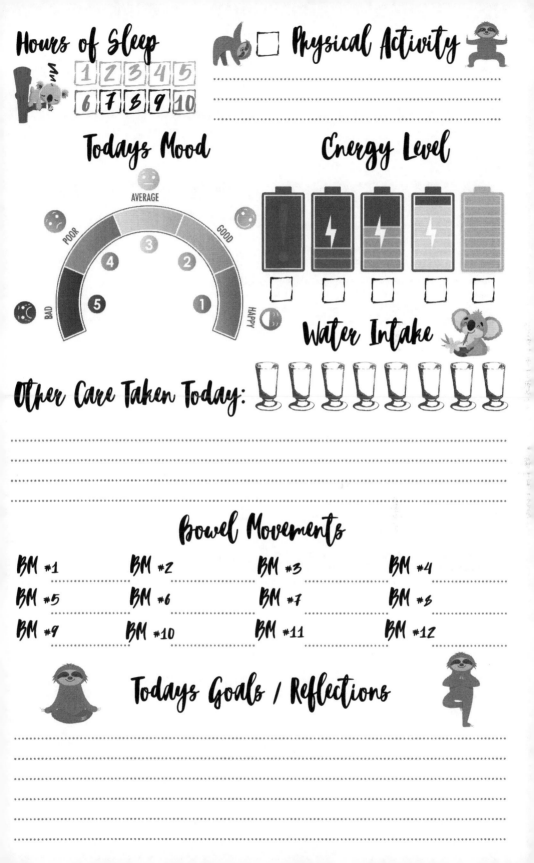

| 1 | 2 | 3 | 4 | 5 |
| 6 | 7 | 8 | 9 | 10 |

☐ Physical Activity

....
....
....

Todays Mood

AVERAGE

POOR

GOOD

3

4

2

BAD

5

1

HAPPY

Energy Level

☐ ☐ ☐ ☐ ☐

Water Intake

Other Care Taken Today:

....
....
....
....

Bowel Movements

BM #1	BM #2	BM #3	BM #4
BM #5	BM #6	BM #7	BM #8
BM #9	BM #10	BM #11	BM #12

Todays Goals / Reflections

....
....
....
....
....
....

DATE _____   **WEIGHT** _____

BREAKFAST

....
....
....
....

TIME _____

PAIN LEVEL (1) (2) (3) (4) (5) (6) (7) (8) (9) (10)

SYMPTOMS

- ☐ BLOODY STOOLS
- ☐ ABDOMINAL PAIN
- ☐ REDUCED APPETITE
- ☐ ....
- ☐ DIARRHEA
- ☐ FATIGUE
- ☐ WEIGHT LOSS
- ☐ ....

LUNCH

....
....
....
....

TIME _____

PAIN LEVEL (1) (2) (3) (4) (5) (6) (7) (8) (9) (10)

SYMPTOMS

- ☐ BLOODY STOOLS
- ☐ ABDOMINAL PAIN
- ☐ REDUCED APPETITE
- ☐ ....
- ☐ DIARRHEA
- ☐ FATIGUE
- ☐ WEIGHT LOSS
- ☐ ....

DINNER

....
....
....
....

TIME _____

PAIN LEVEL (1) (2) (3) (4) (5) (6) (7) (8) (9) (10)

SYMPTOMS

- ☐ BLOODY STOOLS
- ☐ ABDOMINAL PAIN
- ☐ REDUCED APPETITE
- ☐ ....
- ☐ DIARRHEA
- ☐ FATIGUE
- ☐ WEIGHT LOSS
- ☐ ....

SNACKS

....
....
....
....

TIME _____

PAIN LEVEL (1) (2) (3) (4) (5) (6) (7) (8) (9) (10)

SYMPTOMS

- ☐ BLOODY STOOLS
- ☐ ABDOMINAL PAIN
- ☐ REDUCED APPETITE
- ☐ ....
- ☐ DIARRHEA
- ☐ FATIGUE
- ☐ WEIGHT LOSS
- ☐ ....

SNACKS

....
....
....
....

TIME _____

PAIN LEVEL (1) (2) (3) (4) (5) (6) (7) (8) (9) (10)

SYMPTOMS

- ☐ BLOODY STOOLS
- ☐ ABDOMINAL PAIN
- ☐ REDUCED APPETITE
- ☐ ....
- ☐ DIARRHEA
- ☐ FATIGUE
- ☐ WEIGHT LOSS
- ☐ ....

MEDICATIONS & SUPPLEMENTS

....
....
....
....
....
....
....
....
....

EXTRA NOTES

....
....
....
....
....
....
....
....
....

Hours of Sleep

| 1 | 2 | 3 | 4 | 5 |
| 6 | 7 | 8 | 9 | 10 |

Physical Activity

....
....
....

Todays Mood

AVERAGE
POOR
GOOD
BAD
HAPPY

3
4
2
5
1

Energy Level

☐ ☐ ☐ ☐ ☐

Water Intake

Other Care Taken Today:

....
....
....
....

Bowel Movements

BM #1	BM #2	BM #3	BM #4
BM #5	BM #6	BM #7	BM #8
BM #9	BM #10	BM #11	BM #12

Todays Goals / Reflections

....
....
....
....
....

DATE _____   **WEIGHT** _____

BREAKFAST

....
....
....
....

TIME _____

PAIN LEVEL (1) (2) (3) (4) (5) (6) (7) (8) (9) (10)

SYMPTOMS

☐ BLOODY STOOLS   ☐ DIARRHEA

☐ ABDOMINAL PAIN   ☐ FATIGUE

☐ REDUCED APPETITE   ☐ WEIGHT LOSS

☐ ....   ☐ ....

LUNCH

....
....
....
....

TIME _____

PAIN LEVEL (1) (2) (3) (4) (5) (6) (7) (8) (9) (10)

SYMPTOMS

☐ BLOODY STOOLS   ☐ DIARRHEA

☐ ABDOMINAL PAIN   ☐ FATIGUE

☐ REDUCED APPETITE   ☐ WEIGHT LOSS

☐ ....   ☐ ....

DINNER

....
....
....
....

TIME _____

PAIN LEVEL (1) (2) (3) (4) (5) (6) (7) (8) (9) (10)

SYMPTOMS

☐ BLOODY STOOLS   ☐ DIARRHEA

☐ ABDOMINAL PAIN   ☐ FATIGUE

☐ REDUCED APPETITE   ☐ WEIGHT LOSS

☐ ....   ☐ ....

SNACKS

....
....
....
....

TIME _____

PAIN LEVEL (1) (2) (3) (4) (5) (6) (7) (8) (9) (10)

SYMPTOMS

☐ BLOODY STOOLS   ☐ DIARRHEA

☐ ABDOMINAL PAIN   ☐ FATIGUE

☐ REDUCED APPETITE   ☐ WEIGHT LOSS

☐ ....   ☐ ....

SNACKS

....
....
....
....

TIME _____

PAIN LEVEL (1) (2) (3) (4) (5) (6) (7) (8) (9) (10)

SYMPTOMS

☐ BLOODY STOOLS   ☐ DIARRHEA

☐ ABDOMINAL PAIN   ☐ FATIGUE

☐ REDUCED APPETITE   ☐ WEIGHT LOSS

☐ ....   ☐ ....

MEDICATIONS & SUPPLEMENTS

....
....
....
....
....
....
....
....
....
....

EXTRA NOTES

....
....
....
....
....
....
....
....
....
....

Hours of Sleep

| 1 | 2 | 3 | 4 | 5 |
| 6 | 7 | 8 | 9 | 10 |

☐ Physical Activity

....
....
....

Todays Mood

POOR

AVERAGE

GOOD

BAD

HAPPY

3

4

2

5

1

Energy Level

☐ ☐ ☐ ☐ ☐

Water Intake

Other Care Taken Today:

....
....
....
....

Bowel Movements

BM #1	BM #2	BM #3	BM #4
BM #5	BM #6	BM #7	BM #8
BM #9	BM #10	BM #11	BM #12

Todays Goals / Reflections

....
....
....
....
....

DATE _____ **WEIGHT** _____

BREAKFAST

....
....
....

TIME _____

PAIN LEVEL ① ② ③ ④ ⑤ ⑥ ⑦ ⑧ ⑨ ⑩

SYMPTOMS

☐ BLOODY STOOLS ☐ DIARRHEA
☐ ABDOMINAL PAIN ☐ FATIGUE
☐ REDUCED APPETITE ☐ WEIGHT LOSS
☐ .... ☐ ....

LUNCH

....
....
....

TIME _____

PAIN LEVEL ① ② ③ ④ ⑤ ⑥ ⑦ ⑧ ⑨ ⑩

SYMPTOMS

☐ BLOODY STOOLS ☐ DIARRHEA
☐ ABDOMINAL PAIN ☐ FATIGUE
☐ REDUCED APPETITE ☐ WEIGHT LOSS
☐ .... ☐ ....

DINNER

....
....
....

TIME _____

PAIN LEVEL ① ② ③ ④ ⑤ ⑥ ⑦ ⑧ ⑨ ⑩

SYMPTOMS

☐ BLOODY STOOLS ☐ DIARRHEA
☐ ABDOMINAL PAIN ☐ FATIGUE
☐ REDUCED APPETITE ☐ WEIGHT LOSS
☐ .... ☐ ....

SNACKS

....
....
....

TIME _____

PAIN LEVEL ① ② ③ ④ ⑤ ⑥ ⑦ ⑧ ⑨ ⑩

SYMPTOMS

☐ BLOODY STOOLS ☐ DIARRHEA
☐ ABDOMINAL PAIN ☐ FATIGUE
☐ REDUCED APPETITE ☐ WEIGHT LOSS
☐ .... ☐ ....

SNACKS

....
....
....

TIME _____

PAIN LEVEL ① ② ③ ④ ⑤ ⑥ ⑦ ⑧ ⑨ ⑩

SYMPTOMS

☐ BLOODY STOOLS ☐ DIARRHEA
☐ ABDOMINAL PAIN ☐ FATIGUE
☐ REDUCED APPETITE ☐ WEIGHT LOSS
☐ .... ☐ ....

MEDICATIONS & SUPPLEMENTS

....
....
....
....
....
....
....
....
....
....

EXTRA NOTES

....
....
....
....
....
....
....
....
....
....

Hours of Sleep

| 1 | 2 | 3 | 4 | 5 |
| 6 | 7 | 8 | 9 | 10 |

Physical Activity

....

....

....

Todays Mood

POOR

AVERAGE

GOOD

BAD

HAPPY

3

4

2

5

1

Energy Level

☐ ☐ ☐ ☐ ☐

Water Intake

Other Care Taken Today:

....

....

....

....

Bowel Movements

BM #1	BM #2	BM #3	BM #4
BM #5	BM #6	BM #7	BM #8
BM #9	BM #10	BM #11	BM #12

Todays Goals / Reflections

....

....

....

....

....

....

DATE _____   **WEIGHT** _____

BREAKFAST

....
....
....
....

TIME _____

PAIN LEVEL ① ② ③ ④ ⑤ ⑥ ⑦ ⑧ ⑨ ⑩

SYMPTOMS

☐ BLOODY STOOLS ☐ DIARRHEA
☐ ABDOMINAL PAIN ☐ FATIGUE
☐ REDUCED APPETITE ☐ WEIGHT LOSS
☐ .... ☐ ....

LUNCH

....
....
....
....

TIME _____

PAIN LEVEL ① ② ③ ④ ⑤ ⑥ ⑦ ⑧ ⑨ ⑩

SYMPTOMS

☐ BLOODY STOOLS ☐ DIARRHEA
☐ ABDOMINAL PAIN ☐ FATIGUE
☐ REDUCED APPETITE ☐ WEIGHT LOSS
☐ .... ☐ ....

DINNER

....
....
....
....

TIME _____

PAIN LEVEL ① ② ③ ④ ⑤ ⑥ ⑦ ⑧ ⑨ ⑩

SYMPTOMS

☐ BLOODY STOOLS ☐ DIARRHEA
☐ ABDOMINAL PAIN ☐ FATIGUE
☐ REDUCED APPETITE ☐ WEIGHT LOSS
☐ .... ☐ ....

SNACKS

....
....
....
....

TIME _____

PAIN LEVEL ① ② ③ ④ ⑤ ⑥ ⑦ ⑧ ⑨ ⑩

SYMPTOMS

☐ BLOODY STOOLS ☐ DIARRHEA
☐ ABDOMINAL PAIN ☐ FATIGUE
☐ REDUCED APPETITE ☐ WEIGHT LOSS
☐ .... ☐ ....

SNACKS

....
....
....
....

TIME _____

PAIN LEVEL ① ② ③ ④ ⑤ ⑥ ⑦ ⑧ ⑨ ⑩

SYMPTOMS

☐ BLOODY STOOLS ☐ DIARRHEA
☐ ABDOMINAL PAIN ☐ FATIGUE
☐ REDUCED APPETITE ☐ WEIGHT LOSS
☐ .... ☐ ....

MEDICATIONS & SUPPLEMENTS

....
....
....
....
....
....
....
....
....
....

EXTRA NOTES

....
....
....
....
....
....
....
....
....
....

Hours of Sleep

| 1 | 2 | 3 | 4 | 5 |
| 6 | 7 | 8 | 9 | 10 |

Physical Activity

☐

....
....
....

Todays Mood

POOR
AVERAGE
GOOD
BAD
HAPPY

3
4
2
5
1

Energy Level

☐ ☐ ☐ ☐ ☐

Water Intake

Other Care Taken Today:

....
....
....
....

Bowel Movements

BM #1	BM #2	BM #3	BM #4
BM #5	BM #6	BM #7	BM #8
BM #9	BM #10	BM #11	BM #12

Todays Goals / Reflections

....
....
....
....
....
....

DATE _____   **WEIGHT** _____

BREAKFAST

....
....
....
....

TIME _____

PAIN LEVEL (1) (2) (3) (4) (5) (6) (7) (8) (9) (10)

SYMPTOMS

☐ BLOODY STOOLS   ☐ DIARRHEA

☐ ABDOMINAL PAIN   ☐ FATIGUE

☐ REDUCED APPETITE ☐ WEIGHT LOSS

☐ .... ☐ ....

LUNCH

....
....
....
....

TIME _____

PAIN LEVEL (1) (2) (3) (4) (5) (6) (7) (8) (9) (10)

SYMPTOMS

☐ BLOODY STOOLS   ☐ DIARRHEA

☐ ABDOMINAL PAIN   ☐ FATIGUE

☐ REDUCED APPETITE ☐ WEIGHT LOSS

☐ .... ☐ ....

DINNER

....
....
....
....

TIME _____

PAIN LEVEL (1) (2) (3) (4) (5) (6) (7) (8) (9) (10)

SYMPTOMS

☐ BLOODY STOOLS   ☐ DIARRHEA

☐ ABDOMINAL PAIN   ☐ FATIGUE

☐ REDUCED APPETITE ☐ WEIGHT LOSS

☐ .... ☐ ....

SNACKS

....
....
....
....

TIME _____

PAIN LEVEL (1) (2) (3) (4) (5) (6) (7) (8) (9) (10)

SYMPTOMS

☐ BLOODY STOOLS   ☐ DIARRHEA

☐ ABDOMINAL PAIN   ☐ FATIGUE

☐ REDUCED APPETITE ☐ WEIGHT LOSS

☐ .... ☐ ....

SNACKS

....
....
....
....

TIME _____

PAIN LEVEL (1) (2) (3) (4) (5) (6) (7) (8) (9) (10)

SYMPTOMS

☐ BLOODY STOOLS   ☐ DIARRHEA

☐ ABDOMINAL PAIN   ☐ FATIGUE

☐ REDUCED APPETITE ☐ WEIGHT LOSS

☐ .... ☐ ....

MEDICATIONS & SUPPLEMENTS

....
....
....
....
....
....
....
....
....
....

EXTRA NOTES

....
....
....
....
....
....
....
....
....
....

Hours of Sleep

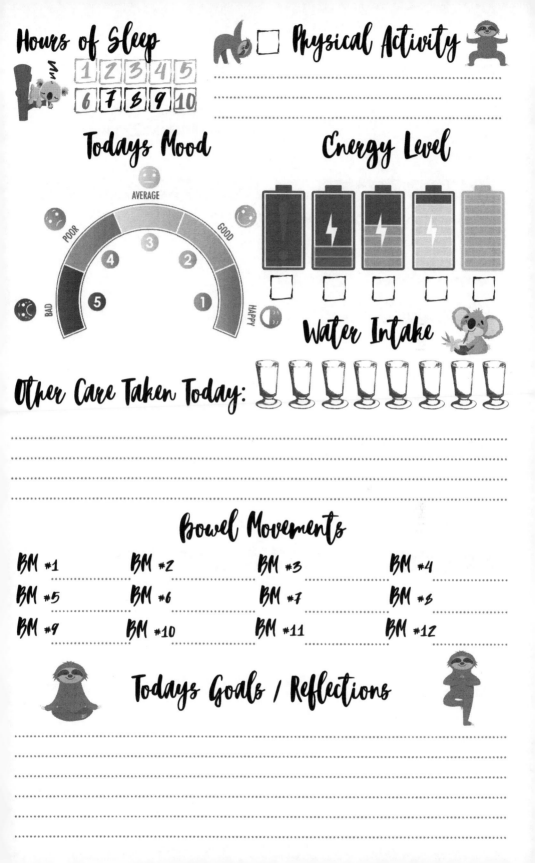

| 1 | 2 | 3 | 4 | 5 |
| 6 | 7 | 8 | 9 | 10 |

Physical Activity

☐

....
....

Todays Mood

POOR

AVERAGE

GOOD

BAD

HAPPY

3

4

2

5

1

Energy Level

☐ ☐ ☐ ☐ ☐

Water Intake

Other Care Taken Today:

....
....
....
....

Bowel Movements

BM #1 .... BM #2 .... BM #3 .... BM #4 ....

BM #5 .... BM #6 .... BM #7 .... BM #8 ....

BM #9 .... BM #10 .... BM #11 .... BM #12 ....

Todays Goals / Reflections

....
....
....
....
....
....

DATE .... **WEIGHT** ....

BREAKFAST

....
....
....
....

TIME ....

PAIN LEVEL ① ② ③ ④ ⑤ ⑥ ⑦ ⑧ ⑨ ⑩

SYMPTOMS

☐ BLOODY STOOLS ☐ DIARRHEA

☐ ABDOMINAL PAIN ☐ FATIGUE

☐ REDUCED APPETITE ☐ WEIGHT LOSS

☐ .... ☐ ....

LUNCH

....
....
....
....

TIME ....

PAIN LEVEL ① ② ③ ④ ⑤ ⑥ ⑦ ⑧ ⑨ ⑩

SYMPTOMS

☐ BLOODY STOOLS ☐ DIARRHEA

☐ ABDOMINAL PAIN ☐ FATIGUE

☐ REDUCED APPETITE ☐ WEIGHT LOSS

☐ .... ☐ ....

DINNER

....
....
....
....

TIME ....

PAIN LEVEL ① ② ③ ④ ⑤ ⑥ ⑦ ⑧ ⑨ ⑩

SYMPTOMS

☐ BLOODY STOOLS ☐ DIARRHEA

☐ ABDOMINAL PAIN ☐ FATIGUE

☐ REDUCED APPETITE ☐ WEIGHT LOSS

☐ .... ☐ ....

SNACKS

....
....
....
....

TIME ....

PAIN LEVEL ① ② ③ ④ ⑤ ⑥ ⑦ ⑧ ⑨ ⑩

SYMPTOMS

☐ BLOODY STOOLS ☐ DIARRHEA

☐ ABDOMINAL PAIN ☐ FATIGUE

☐ REDUCED APPETITE ☐ WEIGHT LOSS

☐ .... ☐ ....

SNACKS

....
....
....
....

TIME ....

PAIN LEVEL ① ② ③ ④ ⑤ ⑥ ⑦ ⑧ ⑨ ⑩

SYMPTOMS

☐ BLOODY STOOLS ☐ DIARRHEA

☐ ABDOMINAL PAIN ☐ FATIGUE

☐ REDUCED APPETITE ☐ WEIGHT LOSS

☐ .... ☐ ....

MEDICATIONS & SUPPLEMENTS

....
....
....
....
....
....
....
....
....

EXTRA NOTES

....
....
....
....
....
....
....
....
....

Hours of Sleep

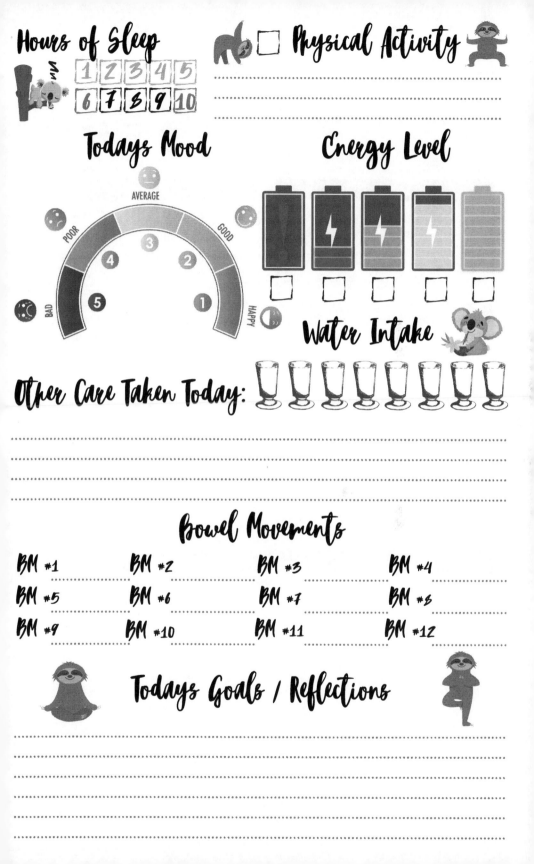

| 1 | 2 | 3 | 4 | 5 |
| 6 | 7 | 8 | 9 | 10 |

Physical Activity

....

....

....

Todays Mood

POOR
AVERAGE
GOOD
BAD
HAPPY

3
4
2
5
1

Energy Level

☐ ☐ ☐ ☐ ☐

Water Intake

Other Care Taken Today:

....

....

....

....

Bowel Movements

BM #1   BM #2   BM #3   BM #4

BM #5   BM #6   BM #7   BM #8

BM #9   BM #10   BM #11   BM #12

Todays Goals / Reflections

....

....

....

....

....

....

DATE .... WEIGHT ....

BREAKFAST

....
....
....
....

TIME ....

PAIN LEVEL ① ② ③ ④ ⑤ ⑥ ⑦ ⑧ ⑨ ⑩

SYMPTOMS

☐ BLOODY STOOLS ☐ DIARRHEA
☐ ABDOMINAL PAIN ☐ FATIGUE
☐ REDUCED APPETITE ☐ WEIGHT LOSS
☐ .... ☐ ....

LUNCH

....
....
....
....

TIME ....

PAIN LEVEL ① ② ③ ④ ⑤ ⑥ ⑦ ⑧ ⑨ ⑩

SYMPTOMS

☐ BLOODY STOOLS ☐ DIARRHEA
☐ ABDOMINAL PAIN ☐ FATIGUE
☐ REDUCED APPETITE ☐ WEIGHT LOSS
☐ .... ☐ ....

DINNER

....
....
....
....

TIME ....

PAIN LEVEL ① ② ③ ④ ⑤ ⑥ ⑦ ⑧ ⑨ ⑩

SYMPTOMS

☐ BLOODY STOOLS ☐ DIARRHEA
☐ ABDOMINAL PAIN ☐ FATIGUE
☐ REDUCED APPETITE ☐ WEIGHT LOSS
☐ .... ☐ ....

SNACKS

....
....
....
....

TIME ....

PAIN LEVEL ① ② ③ ④ ⑤ ⑥ ⑦ ⑧ ⑨ ⑩

SYMPTOMS

☐ BLOODY STOOLS ☐ DIARRHEA
☐ ABDOMINAL PAIN ☐ FATIGUE
☐ REDUCED APPETITE ☐ WEIGHT LOSS
☐ .... ☐ ....

SNACKS

....
....
....
....

TIME ....

PAIN LEVEL ① ② ③ ④ ⑤ ⑥ ⑦ ⑧ ⑨ ⑩

SYMPTOMS

☐ BLOODY STOOLS ☐ DIARRHEA
☐ ABDOMINAL PAIN ☐ FATIGUE
☐ REDUCED APPETITE ☐ WEIGHT LOSS
☐ .... ☐ ....

MEDICATIONS & SUPPLEMENTS

....
....
....
....
....
....
....
....
....
....

EXTRA NOTES

....
....
....
....
....
....
....
....
....
....

Hours of Sleep

1	2	3	4	5
6	7	8	9	10

☐ Physical Activity

....
....
....

Todays Mood

AVERAGE

POOR

GOOD

BAD

HAPPY

3
4
2
5
1

Energy Level

☐ ☐ ☐ ☐ ☐

Water Intake

Other Care Taken Today:

....
....
....
....

Bowel Movements

BM #1 .... BM #2 .... BM #3 .... BM #4 ....

BM #5 .... BM #6 .... BM #7 .... BM #8 ....

BM #9 .... BM #10 .... BM #11 .... BM #12 ....

Todays Goals / Reflections

....
....
....
....
....
....

DATE _____   **WEIGHT** _____

BREAKFAST

....
....
....
....

TIME _____

PAIN LEVEL ① ② ③ ④ ⑤ ⑥ ⑦ ⑧ ⑨ ⑩

SYMPTOMS

☐ BLOODY STOOLS ☐ DIARRHEA
☐ ABDOMINAL PAIN ☐ FATIGUE
☐ REDUCED APPETITE ☐ WEIGHT LOSS
☐ .... ☐ ....

LUNCH

....
....
....
....

TIME _____

PAIN LEVEL ① ② ③ ④ ⑤ ⑥ ⑦ ⑧ ⑨ ⑩

SYMPTOMS

☐ BLOODY STOOLS ☐ DIARRHEA
☐ ABDOMINAL PAIN ☐ FATIGUE
☐ REDUCED APPETITE ☐ WEIGHT LOSS
☐ .... ☐ ....

DINNER

....
....
....
....

TIME _____

PAIN LEVEL ① ② ③ ④ ⑤ ⑥ ⑦ ⑧ ⑨ ⑩

SYMPTOMS

☐ BLOODY STOOLS ☐ DIARRHEA
☐ ABDOMINAL PAIN ☐ FATIGUE
☐ REDUCED APPETITE ☐ WEIGHT LOSS
☐ .... ☐ ....

SNACKS

....
....
....
....

TIME _____

PAIN LEVEL ① ② ③ ④ ⑤ ⑥ ⑦ ⑧ ⑨ ⑩

SYMPTOMS

☐ BLOODY STOOLS ☐ DIARRHEA
☐ ABDOMINAL PAIN ☐ FATIGUE
☐ REDUCED APPETITE ☐ WEIGHT LOSS
☐ .... ☐ ....

SNACKS

....
....
....
....

TIME _____

PAIN LEVEL ① ② ③ ④ ⑤ ⑥ ⑦ ⑧ ⑨ ⑩

SYMPTOMS

☐ BLOODY STOOLS ☐ DIARRHEA
☐ ABDOMINAL PAIN ☐ FATIGUE
☐ REDUCED APPETITE ☐ WEIGHT LOSS
☐ .... ☐ ....

MEDICATIONS & SUPPLEMENTS

....
....
....
....
....
....
....
....
....
....

EXTRA NOTES

....
....
....
....
....
....
....
....
....
....

Hours of Sleep

1 2 3 4 5
6 7 8 9 10

☐ **Physical Activity**

....
....
....

Todays Mood

POOR
AVERAGE
GOOD
BAD
HAPPY
4 3 2 5 1

Energy Level

☐ ☐ ☐ ☐ ☐

Water Intake

Other Care Taken Today:

....
....
....
....

Bowel Movements

BM #1 .... BM #2 .... BM #3 .... BM #4 ....

BM #5 .... BM #6 .... BM #7 .... BM #8 ....

BM #9 .... BM #10 .... BM #11 .... BM #12 ....

Todays Goals / Reflections

....
....
....
....
....

DATE _____ **WEIGHT** _____

BREAKFAST

....
....
....
....

TIME _____

PAIN LEVEL (1)(2)(3)(4)(5)(6)(7)(8)(9)(10)

SYMPTOMS

☐ BLOODY STOOLS ☐ DIARRHEA

☐ ABDOMINAL PAIN ☐ FATIGUE

☐ REDUCED APPETITE ☐ WEIGHT LOSS

☐ .... ☐ ....

LUNCH

....
....
....
....

TIME _____

PAIN LEVEL (1)(2)(3)(4)(5)(6)(7)(8)(9)(10)

SYMPTOMS

☐ BLOODY STOOLS ☐ DIARRHEA

☐ ABDOMINAL PAIN ☐ FATIGUE

☐ REDUCED APPETITE ☐ WEIGHT LOSS

☐ .... ☐ ....

DINNER

....
....
....
....

TIME _____

PAIN LEVEL (1)(2)(3)(4)(5)(6)(7)(8)(9)(10)

SYMPTOMS

☐ BLOODY STOOLS ☐ DIARRHEA

☐ ABDOMINAL PAIN ☐ FATIGUE

☐ REDUCED APPETITE ☐ WEIGHT LOSS

☐ .... ☐ ....

SNACKS

....
....
....
....

TIME _____

PAIN LEVEL (1)(2)(3)(4)(5)(6)(7)(8)(9)(10)

SYMPTOMS

☐ BLOODY STOOLS ☐ DIARRHEA

☐ ABDOMINAL PAIN ☐ FATIGUE

☐ REDUCED APPETITE ☐ WEIGHT LOSS

☐ .... ☐ ....

SNACKS

....
....
....
....

TIME _____

PAIN LEVEL (1)(2)(3)(4)(5)(6)(7)(8)(9)(10)

SYMPTOMS

☐ BLOODY STOOLS ☐ DIARRHEA

☐ ABDOMINAL PAIN ☐ FATIGUE

☐ REDUCED APPETITE ☐ WEIGHT LOSS

☐ .... ☐ ....

MEDICATIONS & SUPPLEMENTS

....
....
....
....
....
....
....
....
....
....

EXTRA NOTES

....
....
....
....
....
....
....
....
....
....

Hours of Sleep

1	2	3	4	5
6	7	8	9	10

Physical Activity ☐

....
....
....

Todays Mood

AVERAGE

POOR

GOOD

3

4 2

BAD

5 1

HAPPY

Energy Level

☐ ☐ ☐ ☐ ☐

Water Intake

Other Care Taken Today:

....
....
....
....

Bowel Movements

BM #1   BM #2   BM #3   BM #4

BM #5   BM #6   BM #7   BM #8

BM #9   BM #10   BM #11   BM #12

Todays Goals / Reflections

....
....
....
....
....
....

DATE _____   **WEIGHT** _____

BREAKFAST

....
....
....
....

TIME _____

PAIN LEVEL ① ② ③ ④ ⑤ ⑥ ⑦ ⑧ ⑨ ⑩

SYMPTOMS

☐ BLOODY STOOLS   ☐ DIARRHEA

☐ ABDOMINAL PAIN   ☐ FATIGUE

☐ REDUCED APPETITE   ☐ WEIGHT LOSS

☐ ....   ☐ ....

LUNCH

....
....
....
....

TIME _____

PAIN LEVEL ① ② ③ ④ ⑤ ⑥ ⑦ ⑧ ⑨ ⑩

SYMPTOMS

☐ BLOODY STOOLS   ☐ DIARRHEA

☐ ABDOMINAL PAIN   ☐ FATIGUE

☐ REDUCED APPETITE   ☐ WEIGHT LOSS

☐ ....   ☐ ....

DINNER

....
....
....
....

TIME _____

PAIN LEVEL ① ② ③ ④ ⑤ ⑥ ⑦ ⑧ ⑨ ⑩

SYMPTOMS

☐ BLOODY STOOLS   ☐ DIARRHEA

☐ ABDOMINAL PAIN   ☐ FATIGUE

☐ REDUCED APPETITE   ☐ WEIGHT LOSS

☐ ....   ☐ ....

SNACKS

....
....
....
....

TIME _____

PAIN LEVEL ① ② ③ ④ ⑤ ⑥ ⑦ ⑧ ⑨ ⑩

SYMPTOMS

☐ BLOODY STOOLS   ☐ DIARRHEA

☐ ABDOMINAL PAIN   ☐ FATIGUE

☐ REDUCED APPETITE   ☐ WEIGHT LOSS

☐ ....   ☐ ....

SNACKS

....
....
....
....

TIME _____

PAIN LEVEL ① ② ③ ④ ⑤ ⑥ ⑦ ⑧ ⑨ ⑩

SYMPTOMS

☐ BLOODY STOOLS   ☐ DIARRHEA

☐ ABDOMINAL PAIN   ☐ FATIGUE

☐ REDUCED APPETITE   ☐ WEIGHT LOSS

☐ ....   ☐ ....

MEDICATIONS & SUPPLEMENTS

....
....
....
....
....
....
....
....
....
....
....

EXTRA NOTES

....
....
....
....
....
....
....
....
....
....
....

Hours of Sleep

1	2	3	4	5
6	7	8	9	10

Physical Activity

☐

....
....

Todays Mood

AVERAGE

POOR

GOOD

3

4   2

BAD

5   1

HAPPY

Energy Level

☐ ☐ ☐ ☐ ☐

Water Intake

Other Care Taken Today:

....
....
....
....

Bowel Movements

BM #1	BM #2	BM #3	BM #4
BM #5	BM #6	BM #7	BM #8
BM #9	BM #10	BM #11	BM #12

Todays Goals / Reflections

....
....
....
....
....

DATE _____ **WEIGHT** _____

BREAKFAST

....
....
....
....

TIME _____

PAIN LEVEL ① ② ③ ④ ⑤ ⑥ ⑦ ⑧ ⑨ ⑩

SYMPTOMS

☐ BLOODY STOOLS   ☐ DIARRHEA
☐ ABDOMINAL PAIN   ☐ FATIGUE
☐ REDUCED APPETITE ☐ WEIGHT LOSS
☐ .... ☐ ....

LUNCH

....
....
....
....

TIME _____

PAIN LEVEL ① ② ③ ④ ⑤ ⑥ ⑦ ⑧ ⑨ ⑩

SYMPTOMS

☐ BLOODY STOOLS   ☐ DIARRHEA
☐ ABDOMINAL PAIN   ☐ FATIGUE
☐ REDUCED APPETITE ☐ WEIGHT LOSS
☐ .... ☐ ....

DINNER

....
....
....
....

TIME _____

PAIN LEVEL ① ② ③ ④ ⑤ ⑥ ⑦ ⑧ ⑨ ⑩

SYMPTOMS

☐ BLOODY STOOLS   ☐ DIARRHEA
☐ ABDOMINAL PAIN   ☐ FATIGUE
☐ REDUCED APPETITE ☐ WEIGHT LOSS
☐ .... ☐ ....

SNACKS

....
....
....
....

TIME _____

PAIN LEVEL ① ② ③ ④ ⑤ ⑥ ⑦ ⑧ ⑨ ⑩

SYMPTOMS

☐ BLOODY STOOLS   ☐ DIARRHEA
☐ ABDOMINAL PAIN   ☐ FATIGUE
☐ REDUCED APPETITE ☐ WEIGHT LOSS
☐ .... ☐ ....

SNACKS

....
....
....
....

TIME _____

PAIN LEVEL ① ② ③ ④ ⑤ ⑥ ⑦ ⑧ ⑨ ⑩

SYMPTOMS

☐ BLOODY STOOLS   ☐ DIARRHEA
☐ ABDOMINAL PAIN   ☐ FATIGUE
☐ REDUCED APPETITE ☐ WEIGHT LOSS
☐ .... ☐ ....

MEDICATIONS & SUPPLEMENTS

....
....
....
....
....
....
....
....
....

EXTRA NOTES

....
....
....
....
....
....
....
....
....
....

Hours of Sleep

| 1 | 2 | 3 | 4 | 5 |
| 6 | 7 | 8 | 9 | 10 |

☐ Physical Activity

....
....
....

Todays Mood

AVERAGE

POOR

GOOD

3

4

2

BAD

5

1

HAPPY

Energy Level

☐ ☐ ☐ ☐ ☐

Water Intake

Other Care Taken Today:

....
....
....
....

Bowel Movements

BM #1 .... BM #2 .... BM #3 .... BM #4 ....

BM #5 .... BM #6 .... BM #7 .... BM #8 ....

BM #9 .... BM #10 .... BM #11 .... BM #12 ....

Todays Goals / Reflections

....
....
....
....
....

DATE _____ **WEIGHT** _____

BREAKFAST

....
....
....
....

TIME _____

PAIN LEVEL ① ② ③ ④ ⑤ ⑥ ⑦ ⑧ ⑨ ⑩

SYMPTOMS

☐ BLOODY STOOLS ☐ DIARRHEA
☐ ABDOMINAL PAIN ☐ FATIGUE
☐ REDUCED APPETITE ☐ WEIGHT LOSS
☐ .... ☐ ....

LUNCH

....
....
....
....

TIME _____

PAIN LEVEL ① ② ③ ④ ⑤ ⑥ ⑦ ⑧ ⑨ ⑩

SYMPTOMS

☐ BLOODY STOOLS ☐ DIARRHEA
☐ ABDOMINAL PAIN ☐ FATIGUE
☐ REDUCED APPETITE ☐ WEIGHT LOSS
☐ .... ☐ ....

DINNER

....
....
....
....

TIME _____

PAIN LEVEL ① ② ③ ④ ⑤ ⑥ ⑦ ⑧ ⑨ ⑩

SYMPTOMS

☐ BLOODY STOOLS ☐ DIARRHEA
☐ ABDOMINAL PAIN ☐ FATIGUE
☐ REDUCED APPETITE ☐ WEIGHT LOSS
☐ .... ☐ ....

SNACKS

....
....
....
....

TIME _____

PAIN LEVEL ① ② ③ ④ ⑤ ⑥ ⑦ ⑧ ⑨ ⑩

SYMPTOMS

☐ BLOODY STOOLS ☐ DIARRHEA
☐ ABDOMINAL PAIN ☐ FATIGUE
☐ REDUCED APPETITE ☐ WEIGHT LOSS
☐ .... ☐ ....

SNACKS

....
....
....
....

TIME _____

PAIN LEVEL ① ② ③ ④ ⑤ ⑥ ⑦ ⑧ ⑨ ⑩

SYMPTOMS

☐ BLOODY STOOLS ☐ DIARRHEA
☐ ABDOMINAL PAIN ☐ FATIGUE
☐ REDUCED APPETITE ☐ WEIGHT LOSS
☐ .... ☐ ....

MEDICATIONS & SUPPLEMENTS

....
....
....
....
....
....
....
....
....
....

EXTRA NOTES

....
....
....
....
....
....
....
....
....
....

Hours of Sleep

| 1 | 2 | 3 | 4 | 5 |
| 6 | 7 | 8 | 9 | 10 |

Physical Activity

....

....

....

Todays Mood

AVERAGE

POOR

GOOD

3

4

2

BAD

5

1

HAPPY

Energy Level

☐ ☐ ☐ ☐ ☐

Water Intake

Other Care Taken Today:

....

....

....

....

Bowel Movements

BM #1   BM #2   BM #3   BM #4

BM #5   BM #6   BM #7   BM #8

BM #9   BM #10   BM #11   BM #12

Todays Goals / Reflections

....

....

....

....

....

....

DATE _____ **WEIGHT** _____

BREAKFAST

....
....
....
....

TIME _____

PAIN LEVEL ① ② ③ ④ ⑤ ⑥ ⑦ ⑧ ⑨ ⑩

SYMPTOMS

☐ BLOODY STOOLS ☐ DIARRHEA
☐ ABDOMINAL PAIN ☐ FATIGUE
☐ REDUCED APPETITE ☐ WEIGHT LOSS
☐ .... ☐ ....

LUNCH

....
....
....
....

TIME _____

PAIN LEVEL ① ② ③ ④ ⑤ ⑥ ⑦ ⑧ ⑨ ⑩

SYMPTOMS

☐ BLOODY STOOLS ☐ DIARRHEA
☐ ABDOMINAL PAIN ☐ FATIGUE
☐ REDUCED APPETITE ☐ WEIGHT LOSS
☐ .... ☐ ....

DINNER

....
....
....
....

TIME _____

PAIN LEVEL ① ② ③ ④ ⑤ ⑥ ⑦ ⑧ ⑨ ⑩

SYMPTOMS

☐ BLOODY STOOLS ☐ DIARRHEA
☐ ABDOMINAL PAIN ☐ FATIGUE
☐ REDUCED APPETITE ☐ WEIGHT LOSS
☐ .... ☐ ....

SNACKS

....
....
....
....

TIME _____

PAIN LEVEL ① ② ③ ④ ⑤ ⑥ ⑦ ⑧ ⑨ ⑩

SYMPTOMS

☐ BLOODY STOOLS ☐ DIARRHEA
☐ ABDOMINAL PAIN ☐ FATIGUE
☐ REDUCED APPETITE ☐ WEIGHT LOSS
☐ .... ☐ ....

SNACKS

....
....
....
....

TIME _____

PAIN LEVEL ① ② ③ ④ ⑤ ⑥ ⑦ ⑧ ⑨ ⑩

SYMPTOMS

☐ BLOODY STOOLS ☐ DIARRHEA
☐ ABDOMINAL PAIN ☐ FATIGUE
☐ REDUCED APPETITE ☐ WEIGHT LOSS
☐ .... ☐ ....

MEDICATIONS & SUPPLEMENTS

....
....
....
....
....
....
....
....
....
....
....

EXTRA NOTES

....
....
....
....
....
....
....
....
....
....
....

Hours of Sleep

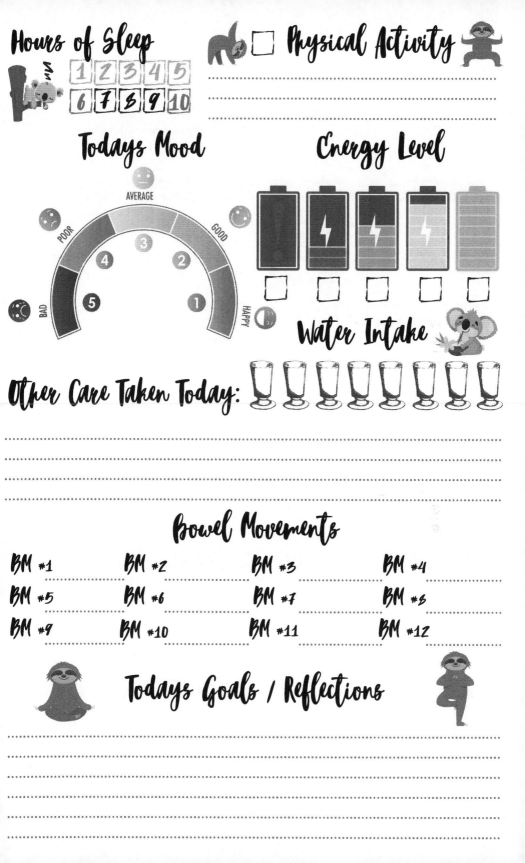

| 1 | 2 | 3 | 4 | 5 |
| 6 | 7 | 8 | 9 | 10 |

Physical Activity

....
....
....

Todays Mood

AVERAGE

POOR

GOOD

3

4

2

5

1

BAD

HAPPY

Energy Level

☐   ☐   ☐   ☐   ☐

Water Intake

Other Care Taken Today:

....
....
....
....

Bowel Movements

BM #1	BM #2	BM #3	BM #4
BM #5	BM #6	BM #7	BM #8
BM #9	BM #10	BM #11	BM #12

Todays Goals / Reflections

....
....
....
....
....

DATE _____ **WEIGHT** _____

BREAKFAST

....
....
....

TIME _____

PAIN LEVEL ① ② ③ ④ ⑤ ⑥ ⑦ ⑧ ⑨ ⑩

SYMPTOMS

☐ BLOODY STOOLS   ☐ DIARRHEA
☐ ABDOMINAL PAIN   ☐ FATIGUE
☐ REDUCED APPETITE   ☐ WEIGHT LOSS
☐ ....   ☐ ....

LUNCH

....
....
....

TIME _____

PAIN LEVEL ① ② ③ ④ ⑤ ⑥ ⑦ ⑧ ⑨ ⑩

SYMPTOMS

☐ BLOODY STOOLS   ☐ DIARRHEA
☐ ABDOMINAL PAIN   ☐ FATIGUE
☐ REDUCED APPETITE   ☐ WEIGHT LOSS
☐ ....   ☐ ....

DINNER

....
....
....

TIME _____

PAIN LEVEL ① ② ③ ④ ⑤ ⑥ ⑦ ⑧ ⑨ ⑩

SYMPTOMS

☐ BLOODY STOOLS   ☐ DIARRHEA
☐ ABDOMINAL PAIN   ☐ FATIGUE
☐ REDUCED APPETITE   ☐ WEIGHT LOSS
☐ ....   ☐ ....

SNACKS

....
....
....

TIME _____

PAIN LEVEL ① ② ③ ④ ⑤ ⑥ ⑦ ⑧ ⑨ ⑩

SYMPTOMS

☐ BLOODY STOOLS   ☐ DIARRHEA
☐ ABDOMINAL PAIN   ☐ FATIGUE
☐ REDUCED APPETITE   ☐ WEIGHT LOSS
☐ ....   ☐ ....

SNACKS

....
....
....

TIME _____

PAIN LEVEL ① ② ③ ④ ⑤ ⑥ ⑦ ⑧ ⑨ ⑩

SYMPTOMS

☐ BLOODY STOOLS   ☐ DIARRHEA
☐ ABDOMINAL PAIN   ☐ FATIGUE
☐ REDUCED APPETITE   ☐ WEIGHT LOSS
☐ ....   ☐ ....

MEDICATIONS & SUPPLEMENTS

....
....
....
....
....
....
....
....

EXTRA NOTES

....
....
....
....
....
....
....
....
....

Hours of Sleep

| 1 | 2 | 3 | 4 | 5 |
| 6 | 7 | 8 | 9 | 10 |

Physical Activity

....
....
....

Todays Mood

AVERAGE

POOR

GOOD

3

4

2

BAD

5

1

HAPPY

Energy Level

☐ ☐ ☐ ☐ ☐

Water Intake

Other Care Taken Today:

....
....
....
....

Bowel Movements

BM #1	BM #2	BM #3	BM #4
BM #5	BM #6	BM #7	BM #8
BM #9	BM #10	BM #11	BM #12

Todays Goals / Reflections

....
....
....
....
....
....

DATE   **WEIGHT**

BREAKFAST

....
....
....
....

TIME

PAIN LEVEL ① ② ③ ④ ⑤ ⑥ ⑦ ⑧ ⑨ ⑩

SYMPTOMS

☐ BLOODY STOOLS   ☐ DIARRHEA

☐ ABDOMINAL PAIN   ☐ FATIGUE

☐ REDUCED APPETITE   ☐ WEIGHT LOSS

☐ ....   ☐ ....

LUNCH

....
....
....
....

TIME

PAIN LEVEL ① ② ③ ④ ⑤ ⑥ ⑦ ⑧ ⑨ ⑩

SYMPTOMS

☐ BLOODY STOOLS   ☐ DIARRHEA

☐ ABDOMINAL PAIN   ☐ FATIGUE

☐ REDUCED APPETITE   ☐ WEIGHT LOSS

☐ ....   ☐ ....

DINNER

....
....
....
....

TIME

PAIN LEVEL ① ② ③ ④ ⑤ ⑥ ⑦ ⑧ ⑨ ⑩

SYMPTOMS

☐ BLOODY STOOLS   ☐ DIARRHEA

☐ ABDOMINAL PAIN   ☐ FATIGUE

☐ REDUCED APPETITE   ☐ WEIGHT LOSS

☐ ....   ☐ ....

SNACKS

....
....
....
....

TIME

PAIN LEVEL ① ② ③ ④ ⑤ ⑥ ⑦ ⑧ ⑨ ⑩

SYMPTOMS

☐ BLOODY STOOLS   ☐ DIARRHEA

☐ ABDOMINAL PAIN   ☐ FATIGUE

☐ REDUCED APPETITE   ☐ WEIGHT LOSS

☐ ....   ☐ ....

SNACKS

....
....
....
....

TIME

PAIN LEVEL ① ② ③ ④ ⑤ ⑥ ⑦ ⑧ ⑨ ⑩

SYMPTOMS

☐ BLOODY STOOLS   ☐ DIARRHEA

☐ ABDOMINAL PAIN   ☐ FATIGUE

☐ REDUCED APPETITE   ☐ WEIGHT LOSS

☐ ....   ☐ ....

MEDICATIONS & SUPPLEMENTS

....
....
....
....
....
....
....
....
....

EXTRA NOTES

....
....
....
....
....
....
....
....
....

Hours of Sleep

1	2	3	4	5
6	7	8	9	10

Physical Activity ☐

....
....
....

Todays Mood

POOR — AVERAGE — GOOD

BAD ... HAPPY

3
4 2
5 1

Energy Level

☐ ☐ ☐ ☐ ☐

Water Intake

Other Care Taken Today:

....
....
....
....

Bowel Movements

BM #1	BM #2	BM #3	BM #4
BM #5	BM #6	BM #7	BM #8
BM #9	BM #10	BM #11	BM #12

Todays Goals / Reflections

....
....
....
....
....
....

DATE _____ **WEIGHT** _____

BREAKFAST

....
....
....

TIME _____

PAIN LEVEL ① ② ③ ④ ⑤ ⑥ ⑦ ⑧ ⑨ ⑩

SYMPTOMS

☐ BLOODY STOOLS   ☐ DIARRHEA

☐ ABDOMINAL PAIN   ☐ FATIGUE

☐ REDUCED APPETITE   ☐ WEIGHT LOSS

☐ ....   ☐ ....

LUNCH

....
....
....

TIME _____

PAIN LEVEL ① ② ③ ④ ⑤ ⑥ ⑦ ⑧ ⑨ ⑩

SYMPTOMS

☐ BLOODY STOOLS   ☐ DIARRHEA

☐ ABDOMINAL PAIN   ☐ FATIGUE

☐ REDUCED APPETITE   ☐ WEIGHT LOSS

☐ ....   ☐ ....

DINNER

....
....
....

TIME _____

PAIN LEVEL ① ② ③ ④ ⑤ ⑥ ⑦ ⑧ ⑨ ⑩

SYMPTOMS

☐ BLOODY STOOLS   ☐ DIARRHEA

☐ ABDOMINAL PAIN   ☐ FATIGUE

☐ REDUCED APPETITE   ☐ WEIGHT LOSS

☐ ....   ☐ ....

SNACKS

....
....
....

TIME _____

PAIN LEVEL ① ② ③ ④ ⑤ ⑥ ⑦ ⑧ ⑨ ⑩

SYMPTOMS

☐ BLOODY STOOLS   ☐ DIARRHEA

☐ ABDOMINAL PAIN   ☐ FATIGUE

☐ REDUCED APPETITE   ☐ WEIGHT LOSS

☐ ....   ☐ ....

SNACKS

....
....
....

TIME _____

PAIN LEVEL ① ② ③ ④ ⑤ ⑥ ⑦ ⑧ ⑨ ⑩

SYMPTOMS

☐ BLOODY STOOLS   ☐ DIARRHEA

☐ ABDOMINAL PAIN   ☐ FATIGUE

☐ REDUCED APPETITE   ☐ WEIGHT LOSS

☐ ....   ☐ ....

MEDICATIONS & SUPPLEMENTS

....
....
....
....
....
....
....

EXTRA NOTES

....
....
....
....
....
....
....

Hours of Sleep

| 1 | 2 | 3 | 4 | 5 |
| 6 | 7 | 8 | 9 | 10 |

☐ Physical Activity

....
....
....

Todays Mood

AVERAGE
POOR
GOOD
BAD
HAPPY

3
4 2
5 1

Energy Level

☐ ☐ ☐ ☐ ☐

Water Intake

Other Care Taken Today:

....
....
....
....

Bowel Movements

BM #1   BM #2   BM #3   BM #4

BM #5   BM #6   BM #7   BM #8

BM #9   BM #10   BM #11   BM #12

Todays Goals / Reflections

....
....
....
....
....

DATE _____ **WEIGHT** _____

BREAKFAST

....
....
....
....

TIME _____

PAIN LEVEL ① ② ③ ④ ⑤ ⑥ ⑦ ⑧ ⑨ ⑩

SYMPTOMS

- ☐ BLOODY STOOLS
- ☐ DIARRHEA
- ☐ ABDOMINAL PAIN
- ☐ FATIGUE
- ☐ REDUCED APPETITE
- ☐ WEIGHT LOSS
- ☐ ....
- ☐ ....

LUNCH

....
....
....
....

TIME _____

PAIN LEVEL ① ② ③ ④ ⑤ ⑥ ⑦ ⑧ ⑨ ⑩

SYMPTOMS

- ☐ BLOODY STOOLS
- ☐ DIARRHEA
- ☐ ABDOMINAL PAIN
- ☐ FATIGUE
- ☐ REDUCED APPETITE
- ☐ WEIGHT LOSS
- ☐ ....
- ☐ ....

DINNER

....
....
....
....

TIME _____

PAIN LEVEL ① ② ③ ④ ⑤ ⑥ ⑦ ⑧ ⑨ ⑩

SYMPTOMS

- ☐ BLOODY STOOLS
- ☐ DIARRHEA
- ☐ ABDOMINAL PAIN
- ☐ FATIGUE
- ☐ REDUCED APPETITE
- ☐ WEIGHT LOSS
- ☐ ....
- ☐ ....

SNACKS

....
....
....
....

TIME _____

PAIN LEVEL ① ② ③ ④ ⑤ ⑥ ⑦ ⑧ ⑨ ⑩

SYMPTOMS

- ☐ BLOODY STOOLS
- ☐ DIARRHEA
- ☐ ABDOMINAL PAIN
- ☐ FATIGUE
- ☐ REDUCED APPETITE
- ☐ WEIGHT LOSS
- ☐ ....
- ☐ ....

SNACKS

....
....
....
....

TIME _____

PAIN LEVEL ① ② ③ ④ ⑤ ⑥ ⑦ ⑧ ⑨ ⑩

SYMPTOMS

- ☐ BLOODY STOOLS
- ☐ DIARRHEA
- ☐ ABDOMINAL PAIN
- ☐ FATIGUE
- ☐ REDUCED APPETITE
- ☐ WEIGHT LOSS
- ☐ ....
- ☐ ....

MEDICATIONS & SUPPLEMENTS

....
....
....
....
....
....
....
....
....
....

EXTRA NOTES

....
....
....
....
....
....
....
....
....
....

Hours of Sleep

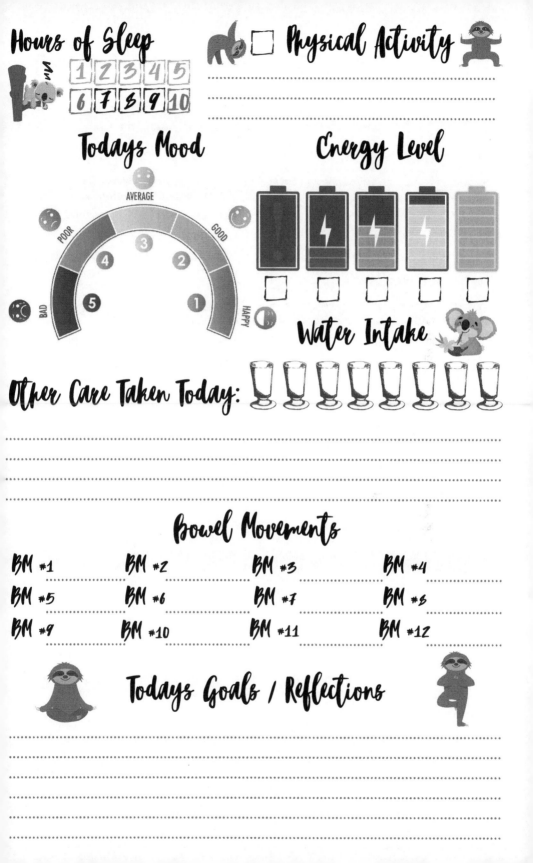

| 1 | 2 | 3 | 4 | 5 |
| 6 | 7 | 8 | 9 | 10 |

Physical Activity

....
....
....

Todays Mood

AVERAGE
POOR
GOOD
3
4 2
BAD 5 1
HAPPY

Energy Level

☐ ☐ ☐ ☐ ☐

Water Intake

Other Care Taken Today:

....
....
....

Bowel Movements

BM #1 .... BM #2 .... BM #3 .... BM #4

BM #5 .... BM #6 .... BM #7 .... BM #8

BM #9 .... BM #10 .... BM #11 .... BM #12

Todays Goals / Reflections

....
....
....
....
....
....

DATE _____ WEIGHT _____

BREAKFAST

....
....
....
....

TIME _____

PAIN LEVEL ① ② ③ ④ ⑤ ⑥ ⑦ ⑧ ⑨ ⑩

SYMPTOMS

☐ BLOODY STOOLS ☐ DIARRHEA
☐ ABDOMINAL PAIN ☐ FATIGUE
☐ REDUCED APPETITE ☐ WEIGHT LOSS
☐ .... ☐ ....

LUNCH

....
....
....
....

TIME _____

PAIN LEVEL ① ② ③ ④ ⑤ ⑥ ⑦ ⑧ ⑨ ⑩

SYMPTOMS

☐ BLOODY STOOLS ☐ DIARRHEA
☐ ABDOMINAL PAIN ☐ FATIGUE
☐ REDUCED APPETITE ☐ WEIGHT LOSS
☐ .... ☐ ....

DINNER

....
....
....
....

TIME _____

PAIN LEVEL ① ② ③ ④ ⑤ ⑥ ⑦ ⑧ ⑨ ⑩

SYMPTOMS

☐ BLOODY STOOLS ☐ DIARRHEA
☐ ABDOMINAL PAIN ☐ FATIGUE
☐ REDUCED APPETITE ☐ WEIGHT LOSS
☐ .... ☐ ....

SNACKS

....
....
....
....

TIME _____

PAIN LEVEL ① ② ③ ④ ⑤ ⑥ ⑦ ⑧ ⑨ ⑩

SYMPTOMS

☐ BLOODY STOOLS ☐ DIARRHEA
☐ ABDOMINAL PAIN ☐ FATIGUE
☐ REDUCED APPETITE ☐ WEIGHT LOSS
☐ .... ☐ ....

SNACKS

....
....
....
....

TIME _____

PAIN LEVEL ① ② ③ ④ ⑤ ⑥ ⑦ ⑧ ⑨ ⑩

SYMPTOMS

☐ BLOODY STOOLS ☐ DIARRHEA
☐ ABDOMINAL PAIN ☐ FATIGUE
☐ REDUCED APPETITE ☐ WEIGHT LOSS
☐ .... ☐ ....

MEDICATIONS & SUPPLEMENTS

....
....
....
....
....
....
....
....
....
....

EXTRA NOTES

....
....
....
....
....
....
....
....
....
....

Hours of Sleep

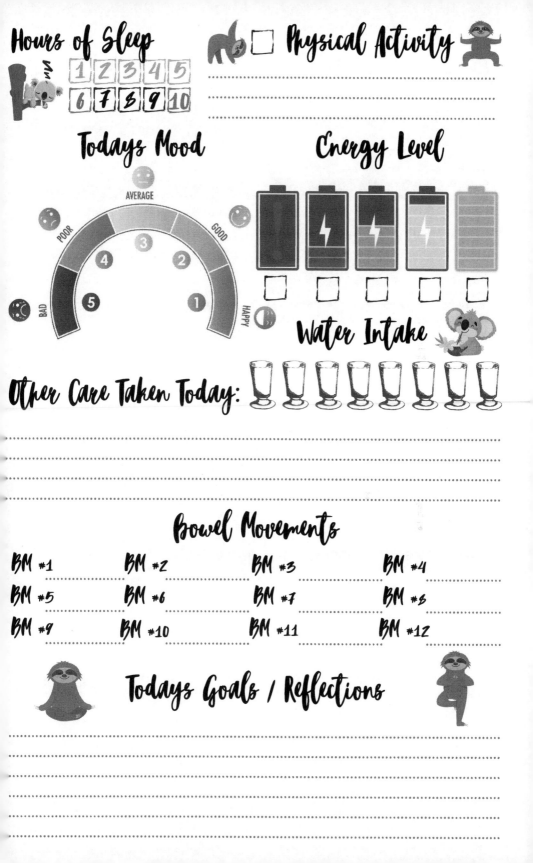

| 1 | 2 | 3 | 4 | 5 |
| 6 | 7 | 8 | 9 | 10 |

Physical Activity

☐

....
....
....

Todays Mood

POOR · AVERAGE · GOOD

4 3 2

5 1

BAD · HAPPY

Energy Level

☐ ☐ ☐ ☐ ☐

Water Intake

Other Care Taken Today:

....
....
....
....

Bowel Movements

BM #1   BM #2   BM #3   BM #4

BM #5   BM #6   BM #7   BM #8

BM #9   BM #10   BM #11   BM #12

Todays Goals / Reflections

....
....
....
....
....

DATE _____ **WEIGHT** _____

BREAKFAST

....
....
....
....

TIME _____

PAIN LEVEL ① ② ③ ④ ⑤ ⑥ ⑦ ⑧ ⑨ ⑩

SYMPTOMS

☐ BLOODY STOOLS   ☐ DIARRHEA
☐ ABDOMINAL PAIN   ☐ FATIGUE
☐ REDUCED APPETITE   ☐ WEIGHT LOSS
☐ ....   ☐ ....

LUNCH

....
....
....
....

TIME _____

PAIN LEVEL ① ② ③ ④ ⑤ ⑥ ⑦ ⑧ ⑨ ⑩

SYMPTOMS

☐ BLOODY STOOLS   ☐ DIARRHEA
☐ ABDOMINAL PAIN   ☐ FATIGUE
☐ REDUCED APPETITE   ☐ WEIGHT LOSS
☐ ....   ☐ ....

DINNER

....
....
....
....

TIME _____

PAIN LEVEL ① ② ③ ④ ⑤ ⑥ ⑦ ⑧ ⑨ ⑩

SYMPTOMS

☐ BLOODY STOOLS   ☐ DIARRHEA
☐ ABDOMINAL PAIN   ☐ FATIGUE
☐ REDUCED APPETITE   ☐ WEIGHT LOSS
☐ ....   ☐ ....

SNACKS

....
....
....
....

TIME _____

PAIN LEVEL ① ② ③ ④ ⑤ ⑥ ⑦ ⑧ ⑨ ⑩

SYMPTOMS

☐ BLOODY STOOLS   ☐ DIARRHEA
☐ ABDOMINAL PAIN   ☐ FATIGUE
☐ REDUCED APPETITE   ☐ WEIGHT LOSS
☐ ....   ☐ ....

SNACKS

....
....
....
....

TIME _____

PAIN LEVEL ① ② ③ ④ ⑤ ⑥ ⑦ ⑧ ⑨ ⑩

SYMPTOMS

☐ BLOODY STOOLS   ☐ DIARRHEA
☐ ABDOMINAL PAIN   ☐ FATIGUE
☐ REDUCED APPETITE   ☐ WEIGHT LOSS
☐ ....   ☐ ....

MEDICATIONS & SUPPLEMENTS

....
....
....
....
....
....
....
....
....
....
....

EXTRA NOTES

....
....
....
....
....
....
....
....
....
....
....

Hours of Sleep

| 1 | 2 | 3 | 4 | 5 |
| 6 | 7 | 8 | 9 | 10 |

Physical Activity

....

....

....

Todays Mood

AVERAGE

POOR

GOOD

BAD

HAPPY

3

4

2

5

1

Energy Level

☐ ☐ ☐ ☐ ☐

Water Intake

Other Care Taken Today:

....

....

....

....

Bowel Movements

BM #1 .... BM #2 .... BM #3 .... BM #4 ....

BM #5 .... BM #6 .... BM #7 .... BM #8 ....

BM #9 .... BM #10 .... BM #11 .... BM #12 ....

Todays Goals / Reflections

....

....

....

....

....

....

DATE _____ **WEIGHT** _____

BREAKFAST

....
....
....
....

TIME _____

PAIN LEVEL ① ② ③ ④ ⑤ ⑥ ⑦ ⑧ ⑨ ⑩

SYMPTOMS

☐ BLOODY STOOLS ☐ DIARRHEA
☐ ABDOMINAL PAIN ☐ FATIGUE
☐ REDUCED APPETITE ☐ WEIGHT LOSS
☐ .... ☐ ....

LUNCH

....
....
....
....

TIME _____

PAIN LEVEL ① ② ③ ④ ⑤ ⑥ ⑦ ⑧ ⑨ ⑩

SYMPTOMS

☐ BLOODY STOOLS ☐ DIARRHEA
☐ ABDOMINAL PAIN ☐ FATIGUE
☐ REDUCED APPETITE ☐ WEIGHT LOSS
☐ .... ☐ ....

DINNER

....
....
....
....

TIME _____

PAIN LEVEL ① ② ③ ④ ⑤ ⑥ ⑦ ⑧ ⑨ ⑩

SYMPTOMS

☐ BLOODY STOOLS ☐ DIARRHEA
☐ ABDOMINAL PAIN ☐ FATIGUE
☐ REDUCED APPETITE ☐ WEIGHT LOSS
☐ .... ☐ ....

SNACKS

....
....
....
....

TIME _____

PAIN LEVEL ① ② ③ ④ ⑤ ⑥ ⑦ ⑧ ⑨ ⑩

SYMPTOMS

☐ BLOODY STOOLS ☐ DIARRHEA
☐ ABDOMINAL PAIN ☐ FATIGUE
☐ REDUCED APPETITE ☐ WEIGHT LOSS
☐ .... ☐ ....

SNACKS

....
....
....
....

TIME _____

PAIN LEVEL ① ② ③ ④ ⑤ ⑥ ⑦ ⑧ ⑨ ⑩

SYMPTOMS

☐ BLOODY STOOLS ☐ DIARRHEA
☐ ABDOMINAL PAIN ☐ FATIGUE
☐ REDUCED APPETITE ☐ WEIGHT LOSS
☐ .... ☐ ....

MEDICATIONS & SUPPLEMENTS

....
....
....
....
....
....
....
....
....
....

EXTRA NOTES

....
....
....
....
....
....
....
....
....
....

Hours of Sleep

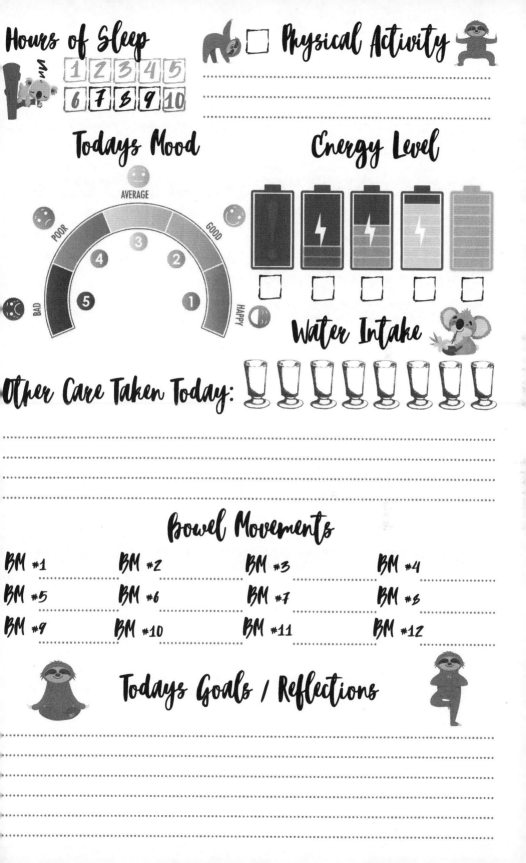

| 1 | 2 | 3 | 4 | 5 |
| 6 | 7 | 8 | 9 | 10 |

☐ Physical Activity

....

....

Todays Mood

AVERAGE

POOR

GOOD

BAD

HAPPY

3

4

2

5

1

Energy Level

☐ ☐ ☐ ☐ ☐

Water Intake

Other Care Taken Today:

....

....

....

....

Bowel Movements

BM #1	BM #2	BM #3	BM #4
BM #5	BM #6	BM #7	BM #8
BM #9	BM #10	BM #11	BM #12

Todays Goals / Reflections

....

....

....

....

....

DATE _____ **WEIGHT** _____

BREAKFAST

....
....
....
....

TIME _____

PAIN LEVEL (1)(2)(3)(4)(5)(6)(7)(8)(9)(10)

SYMPTOMS

- ☐ BLOODY STOOLS
- ☐ DIARRHEA
- ☐ ABDOMINAL PAIN
- ☐ FATIGUE
- ☐ REDUCED APPETITE
- ☐ WEIGHT LOSS
- ☐ .... ☐ ....

LUNCH

....
....
....
....

TIME _____

PAIN LEVEL (1)(2)(3)(4)(5)(6)(7)(8)(9)(10)

SYMPTOMS

- ☐ BLOODY STOOLS
- ☐ DIARRHEA
- ☐ ABDOMINAL PAIN
- ☐ FATIGUE
- ☐ REDUCED APPETITE
- ☐ WEIGHT LOSS
- ☐ .... ☐ ....

DINNER

....
....
....
....

TIME _____

PAIN LEVEL (1)(2)(3)(4)(5)(6)(7)(8)(9)(10)

SYMPTOMS

- ☐ BLOODY STOOLS
- ☐ DIARRHEA
- ☐ ABDOMINAL PAIN
- ☐ FATIGUE
- ☐ REDUCED APPETITE
- ☐ WEIGHT LOSS
- ☐ .... ☐ ....

SNACKS

....
....
....
....

TIME _____

PAIN LEVEL (1)(2)(3)(4)(5)(6)(7)(8)(9)(10)

SYMPTOMS

- ☐ BLOODY STOOLS
- ☐ DIARRHEA
- ☐ ABDOMINAL PAIN
- ☐ FATIGUE
- ☐ REDUCED APPETITE
- ☐ WEIGHT LOSS
- ☐ .... ☐ ....

SNACKS

....
....
....
....

TIME _____

PAIN LEVEL (1)(2)(3)(4)(5)(6)(7)(8)(9)(10)

SYMPTOMS

- ☐ BLOODY STOOLS
- ☐ DIARRHEA
- ☐ ABDOMINAL PAIN
- ☐ FATIGUE
- ☐ REDUCED APPETITE
- ☐ WEIGHT LOSS
- ☐ .... ☐ ....

MEDICATIONS & SUPPLEMENTS

....
....
....
....
....
....
....

EXTRA NOTES

....
....
....
....
....
....
....
....
....
....

Hours of Sleep

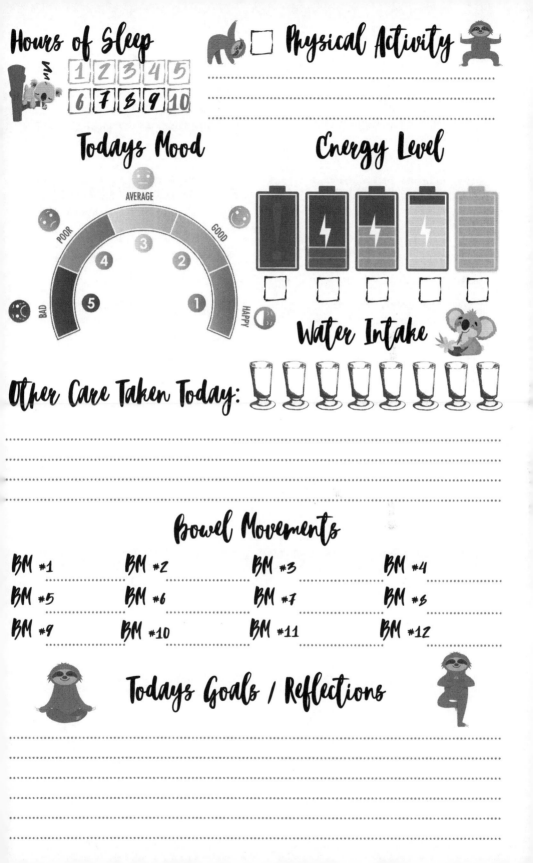

| 1 | 2 | 3 | 4 | 5 |
| 6 | 7 | 8 | 9 | 10 |

Physical Activity

....
....
....

Todays Mood

AVERAGE

POOR

GOOD

3

4

2

BAD

5

1

HAPPY

Energy Level

☐ ☐ ☐ ☐ ☐

Water Intake

Other Care Taken Today:

....
....
....

Bowel Movements

BM #1   BM #2   BM #3   BM #4

BM #5   BM #6   BM #7   BM #8

BM #9   BM #10   BM #11   BM #12

Todays Goals / Reflections

....
....
....
....
....
....

DATE _____   **WEIGHT** _____

BREAKFAST

....
....
....
....

TIME _____

PAIN LEVEL ① ② ③ ④ ⑤ ⑥ ⑦ ⑧ ⑨ ⑩

SYMPTOMS

☐ BLOODY STOOLS ☐ DIARRHEA

☐ ABDOMINAL PAIN ☐ FATIGUE

☐ REDUCED APPETITE ☐ WEIGHT LOSS

☐ .... ☐ ....

LUNCH

....
....
....
....

TIME _____

PAIN LEVEL ① ② ③ ④ ⑤ ⑥ ⑦ ⑧ ⑨ ⑩

SYMPTOMS

☐ BLOODY STOOLS ☐ DIARRHEA

☐ ABDOMINAL PAIN ☐ FATIGUE

☐ REDUCED APPETITE ☐ WEIGHT LOSS

☐ .... ☐ ....

DINNER

....
....
....
....

TIME _____

PAIN LEVEL ① ② ③ ④ ⑤ ⑥ ⑦ ⑧ ⑨ ⑩

SYMPTOMS

☐ BLOODY STOOLS ☐ DIARRHEA

☐ ABDOMINAL PAIN ☐ FATIGUE

☐ REDUCED APPETITE ☐ WEIGHT LOSS

☐ .... ☐ ....

SNACKS

....
....
....
....

TIME _____

PAIN LEVEL ① ② ③ ④ ⑤ ⑥ ⑦ ⑧ ⑨ ⑩

SYMPTOMS

☐ BLOODY STOOLS ☐ DIARRHEA

☐ ABDOMINAL PAIN ☐ FATIGUE

☐ REDUCED APPETITE ☐ WEIGHT LOSS

☐ .... ☐ ....

SNACKS

....
....
....
....

TIME _____

PAIN LEVEL ① ② ③ ④ ⑤ ⑥ ⑦ ⑧ ⑨ ⑩

SYMPTOMS

☐ BLOODY STOOLS ☐ DIARRHEA

☐ ABDOMINAL PAIN ☐ FATIGUE

☐ REDUCED APPETITE ☐ WEIGHT LOSS

☐ .... ☐ ....

MEDICATIONS & SUPPLEMENTS

....
....
....
....
....
....
....
....
....
....

EXTRA NOTES

....
....
....
....
....
....
....
....
....
....

Hours of Sleep

1 2 3 4 5
6 7 8 9 10

Physical Activity

....
....
....

Todays Mood

AVERAGE
POOR
GOOD
3
4 2
BAD
5
1
HAPPY

Energy Level

☐ ☐ ☐ ☐ ☐

Water Intake

Other Care Taken Today:

....
....
....
....

Bowel Movements

BM #1   BM #2   BM #3   BM #4

BM #5   BM #6   BM #7   BM #8

BM #9   BM #10   BM #11   BM #12

Todays Goals / Reflections

....
....
....
....
....
....

DATE ▨▨▨▨▨▨▨▨▨▨▨▨▨ WEIGHT ▨▨▨▨▨▨▨▨▨▨

BREAKFAST

....
....
....
....

TIME ▨▨▨▨▨▨▨▨▨▨▨▨▨▨▨▨▨▨

PAIN LEVEL ① ② ③ ④ ⑤ ⑥ ⑦ ⑧ ⑨ ⑩

SYMPTOMS

☐ BLOODY STOOLS ☐ DIARRHEA
☐ ABDOMINAL PAIN ☐ FATIGUE
☐ REDUCED APPETITE ☐ WEIGHT LOSS
☐ .... ☐ ....

LUNCH

....
....
....
....

TIME ▨▨▨▨▨▨▨▨▨▨▨▨▨▨▨▨▨▨

PAIN LEVEL ① ② ③ ④ ⑤ ⑥ ⑦ ⑧ ⑨ ⑩

SYMPTOMS

☐ BLOODY STOOLS ☐ DIARRHEA
☐ ABDOMINAL PAIN ☐ FATIGUE
☐ REDUCED APPETITE ☐ WEIGHT LOSS
☐ .... ☐ ....

DINNER

....
....
....
....

TIME ▨▨▨▨▨▨▨▨▨▨▨▨▨▨▨▨▨▨

PAIN LEVEL ① ② ③ ④ ⑤ ⑥ ⑦ ⑧ ⑨ ⑩

SYMPTOMS

☐ BLOODY STOOLS ☐ DIARRHEA
☐ ABDOMINAL PAIN ☐ FATIGUE
☐ REDUCED APPETITE ☐ WEIGHT LOSS
☐ .... ☐ ....

SNACKS

....
....
....
....

TIME ▨▨▨▨▨▨▨▨▨▨▨▨▨▨▨▨▨▨

PAIN LEVEL ① ② ③ ④ ⑤ ⑥ ⑦ ⑧ ⑨ ⑩

SYMPTOMS

☐ BLOODY STOOLS ☐ DIARRHEA
☐ ABDOMINAL PAIN ☐ FATIGUE
☐ REDUCED APPETITE ☐ WEIGHT LOSS
☐ .... ☐ ....

SNACKS

....
....
....
....

TIME ▨▨▨▨▨▨▨▨▨▨▨▨▨▨▨▨▨▨

PAIN LEVEL ① ② ③ ④ ⑤ ⑥ ⑦ ⑧ ⑨ ⑩

SYMPTOMS

☐ BLOODY STOOLS ☐ DIARRHEA
☐ ABDOMINAL PAIN ☐ FATIGUE
☐ REDUCED APPETITE ☐ WEIGHT LOSS
☐ .... ☐ ....

MEDICATIONS & SUPPLEMENTS

....
....
....
....
....
....
....
....
....
....
....

EXTRA NOTES

....
....
....
....
....
....
....
....
....
....
....

Hours of Sleep

1	2	3	4	5
6	7	8	9	10

Physical Activity

☐

....
....
....

Todays Mood

AVERAGE

POOR

GOOD

3

4

2

BAD

5

1

HAPPY

Energy Level

☐ ☐ ☐ ☐ ☐

Water Intake

Other Care Taken Today:

....
....
....
....

Bowel Movements

BM #1	BM #2	BM #3	BM #4
BM #5	BM #6	BM #7	BM #8
BM #9	BM #10	BM #11	BM #12

Todays Goals / Reflections

....
....
....
....
....

DATE _____   **WEIGHT** _____

BREAKFAST

....
....
....
....

TIME _____

PAIN LEVEL ① ② ③ ④ ⑤ ⑥ ⑦ ⑧ ⑨ ⑩

SYMPTOMS

☐ BLOODY STOOLS ☐ DIARRHEA
☐ ABDOMINAL PAIN ☐ FATIGUE
☐ REDUCED APPETITE ☐ WEIGHT LOSS
☐ .... ☐ ....

LUNCH

....
....
....
....

TIME _____

PAIN LEVEL ① ② ③ ④ ⑤ ⑥ ⑦ ⑧ ⑨ ⑩

SYMPTOMS

☐ BLOODY STOOLS ☐ DIARRHEA
☐ ABDOMINAL PAIN ☐ FATIGUE
☐ REDUCED APPETITE ☐ WEIGHT LOSS
☐ .... ☐ ....

DINNER

....
....
....
....

TIME _____

PAIN LEVEL ① ② ③ ④ ⑤ ⑥ ⑦ ⑧ ⑨ ⑩

SYMPTOMS

☐ BLOODY STOOLS ☐ DIARRHEA
☐ ABDOMINAL PAIN ☐ FATIGUE
☐ REDUCED APPETITE ☐ WEIGHT LOSS
☐ .... ☐ ....

SNACKS

....
....
....
....

TIME _____

PAIN LEVEL ① ② ③ ④ ⑤ ⑥ ⑦ ⑧ ⑨ ⑩

SYMPTOMS

☐ BLOODY STOOLS ☐ DIARRHEA
☐ ABDOMINAL PAIN ☐ FATIGUE
☐ REDUCED APPETITE ☐ WEIGHT LOSS
☐ .... ☐ ....

SNACKS

....
....
....
....

TIME _____

PAIN LEVEL ① ② ③ ④ ⑤ ⑥ ⑦ ⑧ ⑨ ⑩

SYMPTOMS

☐ BLOODY STOOLS ☐ DIARRHEA
☐ ABDOMINAL PAIN ☐ FATIGUE
☐ REDUCED APPETITE ☐ WEIGHT LOSS
☐ .... ☐ ....

MEDICATIONS & SUPPLEMENTS

....
....
....
....
....
....
....
....
....
....
....

EXTRA NOTES

....
....
....
....
....
....
....
....
....
....
....

Hours of Sleep

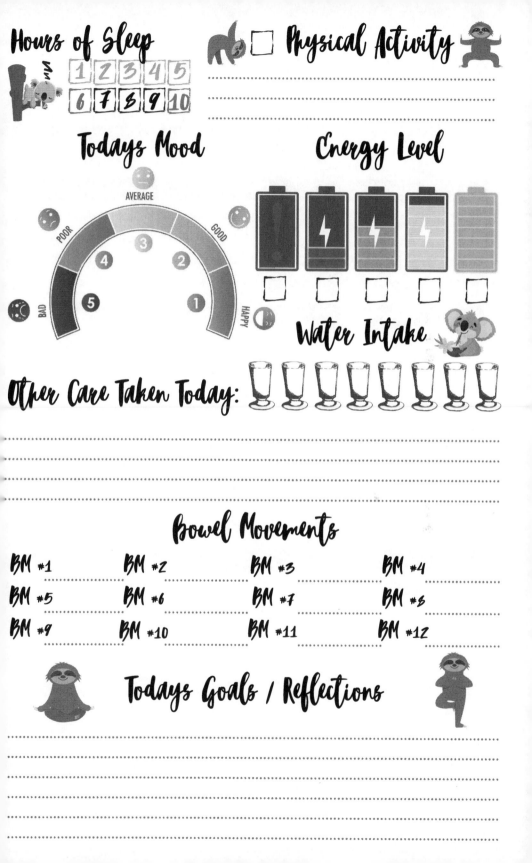

| 1 | 2 | 3 | 4 | 5 |
| 6 | 7 | 8 | 9 | 10 |

Physical Activity

....
....
....

Todays Mood

AVERAGE

POOR

GOOD

4

3

2

5

1

BAD

HAPPY

Energy Level

☐ ☐ ☐ ☐ ☐

Water Intake

Other Care Taken Today:

....
....
....
....

Bowel Movements

BM #1   BM #2   BM #3   BM #4

BM #5   BM #6   BM #7   BM #8

BM #9   BM #10   BM #11   BM #12

Todays Goals / Reflections

....
....
....
....
....

DATE _____ **WEIGHT** _____

BREAKFAST

....
....
....

TIME _____

PAIN LEVEL ① ② ③ ④ ⑤ ⑥ ⑦ ⑧ ⑨ ⑩

SYMPTOMS

☐ BLOODY STOOLS   ☐ DIARRHEA

☐ ABDOMINAL PAIN   ☐ FATIGUE

☐ REDUCED APPETITE   ☐ WEIGHT LOSS

☐ ....   ☐ ....

LUNCH

....
....
....

TIME _____

PAIN LEVEL ① ② ③ ④ ⑤ ⑥ ⑦ ⑧ ⑨ ⑩

SYMPTOMS

☐ BLOODY STOOLS   ☐ DIARRHEA

☐ ABDOMINAL PAIN   ☐ FATIGUE

☐ REDUCED APPETITE   ☐ WEIGHT LOSS

☐ ....   ☐ ....

DINNER

....
....
....

TIME _____

PAIN LEVEL ① ② ③ ④ ⑤ ⑥ ⑦ ⑧ ⑨ ⑩

SYMPTOMS

☐ BLOODY STOOLS   ☐ DIARRHEA

☐ ABDOMINAL PAIN   ☐ FATIGUE

☐ REDUCED APPETITE   ☐ WEIGHT LOSS

☐ ....   ☐ ....

SNACKS

....
....
....

TIME _____

PAIN LEVEL ① ② ③ ④ ⑤ ⑥ ⑦ ⑧ ⑨ ⑩

SYMPTOMS

☐ BLOODY STOOLS   ☐ DIARRHEA

☐ ABDOMINAL PAIN   ☐ FATIGUE

☐ REDUCED APPETITE   ☐ WEIGHT LOSS

☐ ....   ☐ ....

SNACKS

....
....
....

TIME _____

PAIN LEVEL ① ② ③ ④ ⑤ ⑥ ⑦ ⑧ ⑨ ⑩

SYMPTOMS

☐ BLOODY STOOLS   ☐ DIARRHEA

☐ ABDOMINAL PAIN   ☐ FATIGUE

☐ REDUCED APPETITE   ☐ WEIGHT LOSS

☐ ....   ☐ ....

MEDICATIONS & SUPPLEMENTS

....
....
....
....
....
....
....
....
....

EXTRA NOTES

....
....
....
....
....
....
....
....
....

Hours of Sleep

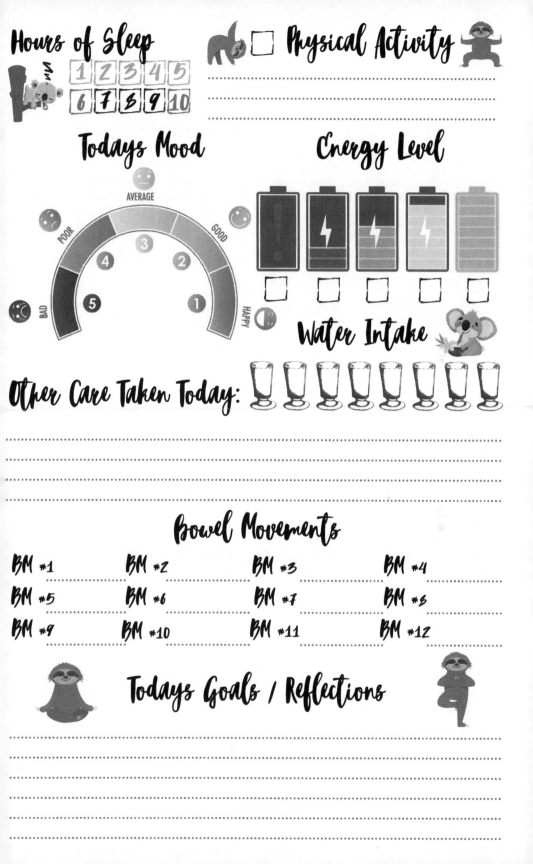

1	2	3	4	5
6	7	8	9	10

Physical Activity

☐

....
....
....

Todays Mood

AVERAGE

POOR

GOOD

3

4   2

BAD   5   1

HAPPY

Energy Level

☐   ☐   ☐   ☐   ☐

Water Intake

Other Care Taken Today:

....
....
....
....

Bowel Movements

BM #1 ....   BM #2 ....   BM #3 ....   BM #4 ....

BM #5 ....   BM #6 ....   BM #7 ....   BM #8 ....

BM #9 ....   BM #10 ....   BM #11 ....   BM #12 ....

Todays Goals / Reflections

....
....
....
....
....
....

DATE _____ **WEIGHT** _____

BREAKFAST

....
....
....
....

TIME _____

PAIN LEVEL (1) (2) (3) (4) (5) (6) (7) (8) (9) (10)

SYMPTOMS

☐ BLOODY STOOLS ☐ DIARRHEA
☐ ABDOMINAL PAIN ☐ FATIGUE
☐ REDUCED APPETITE ☐ WEIGHT LOSS
☐ .... ☐ ....

LUNCH

....
....
....
....

TIME _____

PAIN LEVEL (1) (2) (3) (4) (5) (6) (7) (8) (9) (10)

SYMPTOMS

☐ BLOODY STOOLS ☐ DIARRHEA
☐ ABDOMINAL PAIN ☐ FATIGUE
☐ REDUCED APPETITE ☐ WEIGHT LOSS
☐ .... ☐ ....

DINNER

....
....
....
....

TIME _____

PAIN LEVEL (1) (2) (3) (4) (5) (6) (7) (8) (9) (10)

SYMPTOMS

☐ BLOODY STOOLS ☐ DIARRHEA
☐ ABDOMINAL PAIN ☐ FATIGUE
☐ REDUCED APPETITE ☐ WEIGHT LOSS
☐ .... ☐ ....

SNACKS

....
....
....
....

TIME _____

PAIN LEVEL (1) (2) (3) (4) (5) (6) (7) (8) (9) (10)

SYMPTOMS

☐ BLOODY STOOLS ☐ DIARRHEA
☐ ABDOMINAL PAIN ☐ FATIGUE
☐ REDUCED APPETITE ☐ WEIGHT LOSS
☐ .... ☐ ....

SNACKS

....
....
....
....

TIME _____

PAIN LEVEL (1) (2) (3) (4) (5) (6) (7) (8) (9) (10)

SYMPTOMS

☐ BLOODY STOOLS ☐ DIARRHEA
☐ ABDOMINAL PAIN ☐ FATIGUE
☐ REDUCED APPETITE ☐ WEIGHT LOSS
☐ .... ☐ ....

MEDICATIONS & SUPPLEMENTS

....
....
....
....
....
....
....
....
....

EXTRA NOTES

....
....
....
....
....
....
....
....
....

Hours of Sleep

| 1 | 2 | 3 | 4 | 5 |
| 6 | 7 | 8 | 9 | 10 |

Physical Activity

....
....

Todays Mood

POOR

AVERAGE

GOOD

BAD

HAPPY

3

4

2

5

1

Energy Level

☐ ☐ ☐ ☐ ☐

Water Intake

Other Care Taken Today:

....
....
....
....

Bowel Movements

BM #1 .... BM #2 .... BM #3 .... BM #4 ....

BM #5 .... BM #6 .... BM #7 .... BM #8 ....

BM #9 .... BM #10 .... BM #11 .... BM #12 ....

Todays Goals / Reflections

....
....
....
....
....

DATE ⬚⬚⬚⬚⬚⬚⬚⬚⬚⬚⬚⬚⬚⬚⬚⬚⬚⬚⬚⬚⬚⬚ **WEIGHT** ⬚⬚⬚⬚⬚⬚⬚⬚⬚⬚⬚⬚⬚⬚⬚⬚⬚⬚⬚⬚

BREAKFAST

....
....
....
....

TIME ⬚⬚⬚⬚⬚⬚⬚⬚⬚⬚⬚⬚⬚⬚⬚⬚⬚⬚⬚

PAIN LEVEL   ① ② ③ ④ ⑤ ⑥ ⑦ ⑧ ⑨ ⑩

SYMPTOMS

☐ BLOODY STOOLS   ☐ DIARRHEA

☐ ABDOMINAL PAIN   ☐ FATIGUE

☐ REDUCED APPETITE   ☐ WEIGHT LOSS

☐ ....   ☐ ....

LUNCH

....
....
....
....

TIME ⬚⬚⬚⬚⬚⬚⬚⬚⬚⬚⬚⬚⬚⬚⬚⬚⬚⬚⬚

PAIN LEVEL   ① ② ③ ④ ⑤ ⑥ ⑦ ⑧ ⑨ ⑩

SYMPTOMS

☐ BLOODY STOOLS   ☐ DIARRHEA

☐ ABDOMINAL PAIN   ☐ FATIGUE

☐ REDUCED APPETITE   ☐ WEIGHT LOSS

☐ ....   ☐ ....

DINNER

....
....
....
....

TIME ⬚⬚⬚⬚⬚⬚⬚⬚⬚⬚⬚⬚⬚⬚⬚⬚⬚⬚⬚

PAIN LEVEL   ① ② ③ ④ ⑤ ⑥ ⑦ ⑧ ⑨ ⑩

SYMPTOMS

☐ BLOODY STOOLS   ☐ DIARRHEA

☐ ABDOMINAL PAIN   ☐ FATIGUE

☐ REDUCED APPETITE   ☐ WEIGHT LOSS

☐ ....   ☐ ....

SNACKS

....
....
....
....

TIME ⬚⬚⬚⬚⬚⬚⬚⬚⬚⬚⬚⬚⬚⬚⬚⬚⬚⬚⬚

PAIN LEVEL   ① ② ③ ④ ⑤ ⑥ ⑦ ⑧ ⑨ ⑩

SYMPTOMS

☐ BLOODY STOOLS   ☐ DIARRHEA

☐ ABDOMINAL PAIN   ☐ FATIGUE

☐ REDUCED APPETITE   ☐ WEIGHT LOSS

☐ ....   ☐ ....

SNACKS

....
....
....
....

TIME ⬚⬚⬚⬚⬚⬚⬚⬚⬚⬚⬚⬚⬚⬚⬚⬚⬚⬚⬚

PAIN LEVEL   ① ② ③ ④ ⑤ ⑥ ⑦ ⑧ ⑨ ⑩

SYMPTOMS

☐ BLOODY STOOLS   ☐ DIARRHEA

☐ ABDOMINAL PAIN   ☐ FATIGUE

☐ REDUCED APPETITE   ☐ WEIGHT LOSS

☐ ....   ☐ ....

MEDICATIONS & SUPPLEMENTS

....
....
....
....
....
....
....
....
....
....

EXTRA NOTES

....
....
....
....
....
....
....
....
....
....

Hours of Sleep

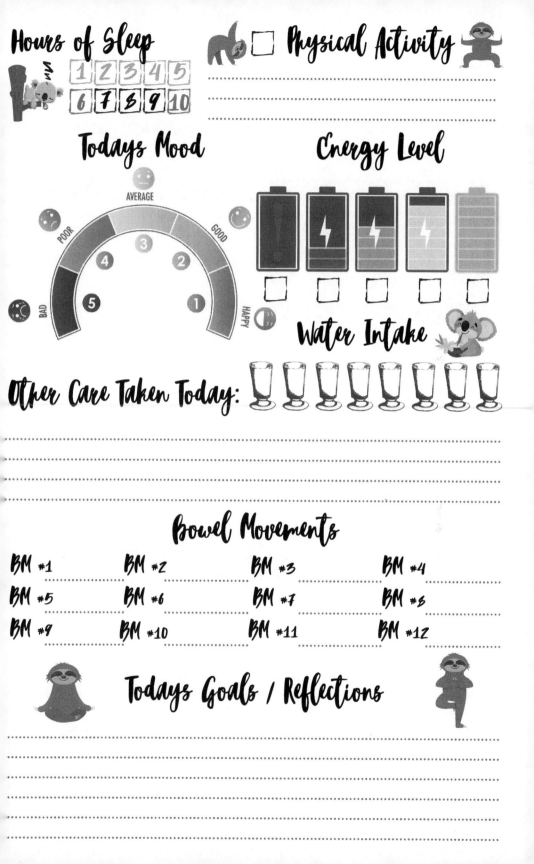

| 1 | 2 | 3 | 4 | 5 |
| 6 | 7 | 8 | 9 | 10 |

☐ Physical Activity

....
....
....

Todays Mood

AVERAGE

POOR

GOOD

BAD

HAPPY

3
4
2
5
1

Energy Level

☐ ☐ ☐ ☐ ☐

Water Intake

Other Care Taken Today:

....
....
....
....

Bowel Movements

BM #1   BM #2   BM #3   BM #4

BM #5   BM #6   BM #7   BM #8

BM #9   BM #10   BM #11   BM #12

Todays Goals / Reflections

....
....
....
....
....

DATE _____ **WEIGHT** _____

BREAKFAST

....
....
....
....

TIME _____

PAIN LEVEL ① ② ③ ④ ⑤ ⑥ ⑦ ⑧ ⑨ ⑩

SYMPTOMS

☐ BLOODY STOOLS ☐ DIARRHEA
☐ ABDOMINAL PAIN ☐ FATIGUE
☐ REDUCED APPETITE ☐ WEIGHT LOSS
☐ .... ☐ ....

LUNCH

....
....
....
....

TIME _____

PAIN LEVEL ① ② ③ ④ ⑤ ⑥ ⑦ ⑧ ⑨ ⑩

SYMPTOMS

☐ BLOODY STOOLS ☐ DIARRHEA
☐ ABDOMINAL PAIN ☐ FATIGUE
☐ REDUCED APPETITE ☐ WEIGHT LOSS
☐ .... ☐ ....

DINNER

....
....
....
....

TIME _____

PAIN LEVEL ① ② ③ ④ ⑤ ⑥ ⑦ ⑧ ⑨ ⑩

SYMPTOMS

☐ BLOODY STOOLS ☐ DIARRHEA
☐ ABDOMINAL PAIN ☐ FATIGUE
☐ REDUCED APPETITE ☐ WEIGHT LOSS
☐ .... ☐ ....

SNACKS

....
....
....
....

TIME _____

PAIN LEVEL ① ② ③ ④ ⑤ ⑥ ⑦ ⑧ ⑨ ⑩

SYMPTOMS

☐ BLOODY STOOLS ☐ DIARRHEA
☐ ABDOMINAL PAIN ☐ FATIGUE
☐ REDUCED APPETITE ☐ WEIGHT LOSS
☐ .... ☐ ....

SNACKS

....
....
....
....

TIME _____

PAIN LEVEL ① ② ③ ④ ⑤ ⑥ ⑦ ⑧ ⑨ ⑩

SYMPTOMS

☐ BLOODY STOOLS ☐ DIARRHEA
☐ ABDOMINAL PAIN ☐ FATIGUE
☐ REDUCED APPETITE ☐ WEIGHT LOSS
☐ .... ☐ ....

MEDICATIONS & SUPPLEMENTS

....
....
....
....
....
....
....
....
....
....
....

EXTRA NOTES

....
....
....
....
....
....
....
....
....
....
....

Hours of Sleep

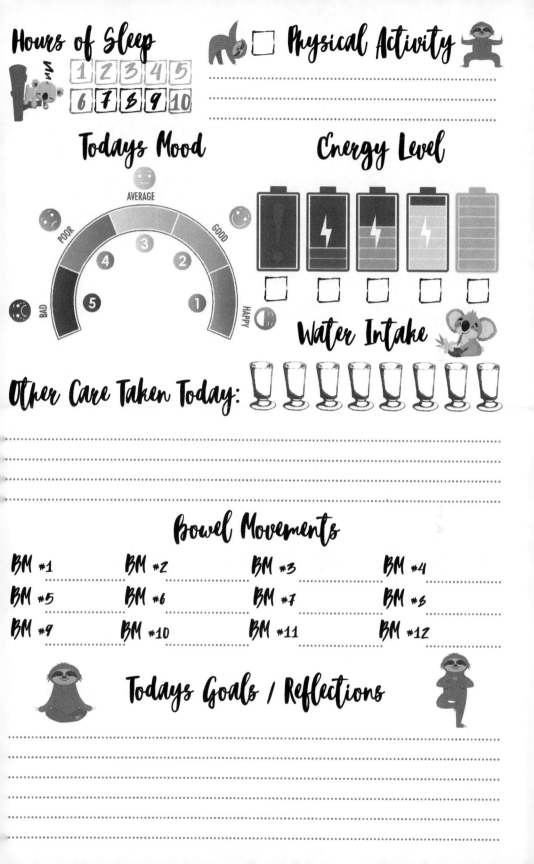

| 1 | 2 | 3 | 4 | 5 |
| 6 | 7 | 8 | 9 | 10 |

Physical Activity

☐

....
....
....

Todays Mood

AVERAGE

POOR

GOOD

3

4

2

5

1

BAD

HAPPY

Energy Level

☐ ☐ ☐ ☐ ☐

Water Intake

Other Care Taken Today:

....
....
....
....

Bowel Movements

BM #1   BM #2   BM #3   BM #4

BM #5   BM #6   BM #7   BM #8

BM #9   BM #10   BM #11   BM #12

Todays Goals / Reflections

....
....
....
....
....

DATE _____ **WEIGHT** _____

BREAKFAST

....
....
....
....

TIME _____

PAIN LEVEL ① ② ③ ④ ⑤ ⑥ ⑦ ⑧ ⑨ ⑩

SYMPTOMS

☐ BLOODY STOOLS ☐ DIARRHEA

☐ ABDOMINAL PAIN ☐ FATIGUE

☐ REDUCED APPETITE ☐ WEIGHT LOSS

☐ .... ☐ ....

LUNCH

....
....
....
....

TIME _____

PAIN LEVEL ① ② ③ ④ ⑤ ⑥ ⑦ ⑧ ⑨ ⑩

SYMPTOMS

☐ BLOODY STOOLS ☐ DIARRHEA

☐ ABDOMINAL PAIN ☐ FATIGUE

☐ REDUCED APPETITE ☐ WEIGHT LOSS

☐ .... ☐ ....

DINNER

....
....
....
....

TIME _____

PAIN LEVEL ① ② ③ ④ ⑤ ⑥ ⑦ ⑧ ⑨ ⑩

SYMPTOMS

☐ BLOODY STOOLS ☐ DIARRHEA

☐ ABDOMINAL PAIN ☐ FATIGUE

☐ REDUCED APPETITE ☐ WEIGHT LOSS

☐ .... ☐ ....

SNACKS

....
....
....
....

TIME _____

PAIN LEVEL ① ② ③ ④ ⑤ ⑥ ⑦ ⑧ ⑨ ⑩

SYMPTOMS

☐ BLOODY STOOLS ☐ DIARRHEA

☐ ABDOMINAL PAIN ☐ FATIGUE

☐ REDUCED APPETITE ☐ WEIGHT LOSS

☐ .... ☐ ....

SNACKS

....
....
....
....

TIME _____

PAIN LEVEL ① ② ③ ④ ⑤ ⑥ ⑦ ⑧ ⑨ ⑩

SYMPTOMS

☐ BLOODY STOOLS ☐ DIARRHEA

☐ ABDOMINAL PAIN ☐ FATIGUE

☐ REDUCED APPETITE ☐ WEIGHT LOSS

☐ .... ☐ ....

MEDICATIONS & SUPPLEMENTS

....
....
....
....
....
....
....
....
....
....

EXTRA NOTES

....
....
....
....
....
....
....
....
....
....

Hours of Sleep

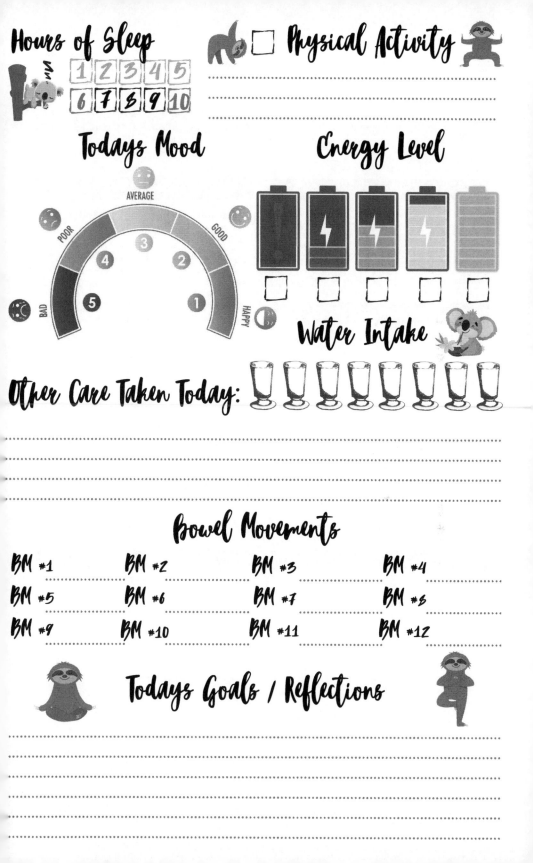

1	2	3	4	5
6	7	8	9	10

Physical Activity

....
....
....

Todays Mood

AVERAGE

POOR

GOOD

3

4

2

BAD

5

1

HAPPY

Energy Level

☐ ☐ ☐ ☐ ☐

Water Intake

Other Care Taken Today:

....
....
....
....

Bowel Movements

BM #1	BM #2	BM #3	BM #4
BM #5	BM #6	BM #7	BM #8
BM #9	BM #10	BM #11	BM #12

Todays Goals / Reflections

....
....
....
....
....

DATE _____   WEIGHT _____

BREAKFAST

....
....
....
....

TIME _____

PAIN LEVEL ① ② ③ ④ ⑤ ⑥ ⑦ ⑧ ⑨ ⑩

SYMPTOMS

☐ BLOODY STOOLS ☐ DIARRHEA

☐ ABDOMINAL PAIN ☐ FATIGUE

☐ REDUCED APPETITE ☐ WEIGHT LOSS

☐ .... ☐ ....

LUNCH

....
....
....
....

TIME _____

PAIN LEVEL ① ② ③ ④ ⑤ ⑥ ⑦ ⑧ ⑨ ⑩

SYMPTOMS

☐ BLOODY STOOLS ☐ DIARRHEA

☐ ABDOMINAL PAIN ☐ FATIGUE

☐ REDUCED APPETITE ☐ WEIGHT LOSS

☐ .... ☐ ....

DINNER

....
....
....
....

TIME _____

PAIN LEVEL ① ② ③ ④ ⑤ ⑥ ⑦ ⑧ ⑨ ⑩

SYMPTOMS

☐ BLOODY STOOLS ☐ DIARRHEA

☐ ABDOMINAL PAIN ☐ FATIGUE

☐ REDUCED APPETITE ☐ WEIGHT LOSS

☐ .... ☐ ....

SNACKS

....
....
....
....

TIME _____

PAIN LEVEL ① ② ③ ④ ⑤ ⑥ ⑦ ⑧ ⑨ ⑩

SYMPTOMS

☐ BLOODY STOOLS ☐ DIARRHEA

☐ ABDOMINAL PAIN ☐ FATIGUE

☐ REDUCED APPETITE ☐ WEIGHT LOSS

☐ .... ☐ ....

SNACKS

....
....
....
....

TIME _____

PAIN LEVEL ① ② ③ ④ ⑤ ⑥ ⑦ ⑧ ⑨ ⑩

SYMPTOMS

☐ BLOODY STOOLS ☐ DIARRHEA

☐ ABDOMINAL PAIN ☐ FATIGUE

☐ REDUCED APPETITE ☐ WEIGHT LOSS

☐ .... ☐ ....

MEDICATIONS & SUPPLEMENTS

....
....
....
....
....
....
....
....
....
....

EXTRA NOTES

....
....
....
....
....
....
....
....
....
....

Hours of Sleep

| 1 | 2 | 3 | 4 | 5 |
| 6 | 7 | 8 | 9 | 10 |

Physical Activity ☐

....
....
....

Todays Mood

POOR • AVERAGE • GOOD

BAD • HAPPY

3
4 • 2
5 • 1

Energy Level

☐ ☐ ☐ ☐ ☐

Water Intake

Other Care Taken Today:

....
....
....
....

Bowel Movements

BM #1	BM #2	BM #3	BM #4
BM #5	BM #6	BM #7	BM #8
BM #9	BM #10	BM #11	BM #12

Todays Goals / Reflections

....
....
....
....
....
....

DATE _____   **WEIGHT** _____

BREAKFAST

....
....
....
....

TIME _____

PAIN LEVEL ① ② ③ ④ ⑤ ⑥ ⑦ ⑧ ⑨ ⑩

SYMPTOMS

- ☐ BLOODY STOOLS
- ☐ DIARRHEA
- ☐ ABDOMINAL PAIN
- ☐ FATIGUE
- ☐ REDUCED APPETITE
- ☐ WEIGHT LOSS
- ☐ ....
- ☐ ....

LUNCH

....
....
....
....

TIME _____

PAIN LEVEL ① ② ③ ④ ⑤ ⑥ ⑦ ⑧ ⑨ ⑩

SYMPTOMS

- ☐ BLOODY STOOLS
- ☐ DIARRHEA
- ☐ ABDOMINAL PAIN
- ☐ FATIGUE
- ☐ REDUCED APPETITE
- ☐ WEIGHT LOSS
- ☐ ....
- ☐ ....

DINNER

....
....
....
....

TIME _____

PAIN LEVEL ① ② ③ ④ ⑤ ⑥ ⑦ ⑧ ⑨ ⑩

SYMPTOMS

- ☐ BLOODY STOOLS
- ☐ DIARRHEA
- ☐ ABDOMINAL PAIN
- ☐ FATIGUE
- ☐ REDUCED APPETITE
- ☐ WEIGHT LOSS
- ☐ ....
- ☐ ....

SNACKS

....
....
....
....

TIME _____

PAIN LEVEL ① ② ③ ④ ⑤ ⑥ ⑦ ⑧ ⑨ ⑩

SYMPTOMS

- ☐ BLOODY STOOLS
- ☐ DIARRHEA
- ☐ ABDOMINAL PAIN
- ☐ FATIGUE
- ☐ REDUCED APPETITE
- ☐ WEIGHT LOSS
- ☐ ....
- ☐ ....

SNACKS

....
....
....
....

TIME _____

PAIN LEVEL ① ② ③ ④ ⑤ ⑥ ⑦ ⑧ ⑨ ⑩

SYMPTOMS

- ☐ BLOODY STOOLS
- ☐ DIARRHEA
- ☐ ABDOMINAL PAIN
- ☐ FATIGUE
- ☐ REDUCED APPETITE
- ☐ WEIGHT LOSS
- ☐ ....
- ☐ ....

MEDICATIONS & SUPPLEMENTS

....
....
....
....
....
....
....
....
....
....

EXTRA NOTES

....
....
....
....
....
....
....
....
....
....

Hours of Sleep

| 1 | 2 | 3 | 4 | 5 |
| 6 | 7 | 8 | 9 | 10 |

☐ Physical Activity

....
....
....

Todays Mood

POOR · AVERAGE · GOOD · BAD · HAPPY

4 · 3 · 2 · 5 · 1

Energy Level

☐ ☐ ☐ ☐ ☐

Water Intake

Other Care Taken Today:

....
....
....
....

Bowel Movements

BM #1   BM #2   BM #3   BM #4

BM #5   BM #6   BM #7   BM #8

BM #9   BM #10   BM #11   BM #12

Todays Goals / Reflections

....
....
....
....
....

DATE _____ WEIGHT _____

BREAKFAST

....
....
....
....

TIME _____

PAIN LEVEL (1)(2)(3)(4)(5)(6)(7)(8)(9)(10)

SYMPTOMS

☐ BLOODY STOOLS   ☐ DIARRHEA
☐ ABDOMINAL PAIN   ☐ FATIGUE
☐ REDUCED APPETITE   ☐ WEIGHT LOSS
☐ ....   ☐ ....

LUNCH

....
....
....
....

TIME _____

PAIN LEVEL (1)(2)(3)(4)(5)(6)(7)(8)(9)(10)

SYMPTOMS

☐ BLOODY STOOLS   ☐ DIARRHEA
☐ ABDOMINAL PAIN   ☐ FATIGUE
☐ REDUCED APPETITE   ☐ WEIGHT LOSS
☐ ....   ☐ ....

DINNER

....
....
....
....

TIME _____

PAIN LEVEL (1)(2)(3)(4)(5)(6)(7)(8)(9)(10)

SYMPTOMS

☐ BLOODY STOOLS   ☐ DIARRHEA
☐ ABDOMINAL PAIN   ☐ FATIGUE
☐ REDUCED APPETITE   ☐ WEIGHT LOSS
☐ ....   ☐ ....

SNACKS

....
....
....
....

TIME _____

PAIN LEVEL (1)(2)(3)(4)(5)(6)(7)(8)(9)(10)

SYMPTOMS

☐ BLOODY STOOLS   ☐ DIARRHEA
☐ ABDOMINAL PAIN   ☐ FATIGUE
☐ REDUCED APPETITE   ☐ WEIGHT LOSS
☐ ....   ☐ ....

SNACKS

....
....
....
....

TIME _____

PAIN LEVEL (1)(2)(3)(4)(5)(6)(7)(8)(9)(10)

SYMPTOMS

☐ BLOODY STOOLS   ☐ DIARRHEA
☐ ABDOMINAL PAIN   ☐ FATIGUE
☐ REDUCED APPETITE   ☐ WEIGHT LOSS
☐ ....   ☐ ....

MEDICATIONS & SUPPLEMENTS

....
....
....
....
....
....
....
....
....
....
....

EXTRA NOTES

....
....
....
....
....
....
....
....
....
....
....

Hours of Sleep

| 1 | 2 | 3 | 4 | 5 |
| 6 | 7 | 8 | 9 | 10 |

Physical Activity

....
....
....

Todays Mood

AVERAGE

POOR

GOOD

3

4

2

BAD

5

1

HAPPY

Energy Level

☐ ☐ ☐ ☐ ☐

Water Intake

Other Care Taken Today:

....
....
....
....

Bowel Movements

BM #1   BM #2   BM #3   BM #4

BM #5   BM #6   BM #7   BM #8

BM #9   BM #10   BM #11   BM #12

Todays Goals / Reflections

....
....
....
....
....

DATE

WEIGHT

BREAKFAST

....
....
....
....

TIME

PAIN LEVEL (1) (2) (3) (4) (5) (6) (7) (8) (9) (10)

SYMPTOMS

☐ BLOODY STOOLS ☐ DIARRHEA

☐ ABDOMINAL PAIN ☐ FATIGUE

☐ REDUCED APPETITE ☐ WEIGHT LOSS

☐ .... ☐ ....

LUNCH

....
....
....
....

TIME

PAIN LEVEL (1) (2) (3) (4) (5) (6) (7) (8) (9) (10)

SYMPTOMS

☐ BLOODY STOOLS ☐ DIARRHEA

☐ ABDOMINAL PAIN ☐ FATIGUE

☐ REDUCED APPETITE ☐ WEIGHT LOSS

☐ .... ☐ ....

DINNER

....
....
....
....

TIME

PAIN LEVEL (1) (2) (3) (4) (5) (6) (7) (8) (9) (10)

SYMPTOMS

☐ BLOODY STOOLS ☐ DIARRHEA

☐ ABDOMINAL PAIN ☐ FATIGUE

☐ REDUCED APPETITE ☐ WEIGHT LOSS

☐ .... ☐ ....

SNACKS

....
....
....
....

TIME

PAIN LEVEL (1) (2) (3) (4) (5) (6) (7) (8) (9) (10)

SYMPTOMS

☐ BLOODY STOOLS ☐ DIARRHEA

☐ ABDOMINAL PAIN ☐ FATIGUE

☐ REDUCED APPETITE ☐ WEIGHT LOSS

☐ .... ☐ ....

SNACKS

....
....
....
....

TIME

PAIN LEVEL (1) (2) (3) (4) (5) (6) (7) (8) (9) (10)

SYMPTOMS

☐ BLOODY STOOLS ☐ DIARRHEA

☐ ABDOMINAL PAIN ☐ FATIGUE

☐ REDUCED APPETITE ☐ WEIGHT LOSS

☐ .... ☐ ....

MEDICATIONS & SUPPLEMENTS

....
....
....
....
....
....
....
....
....

EXTRA NOTES

....
....
....
....
....
....
....
....
....

Hours of Sleep

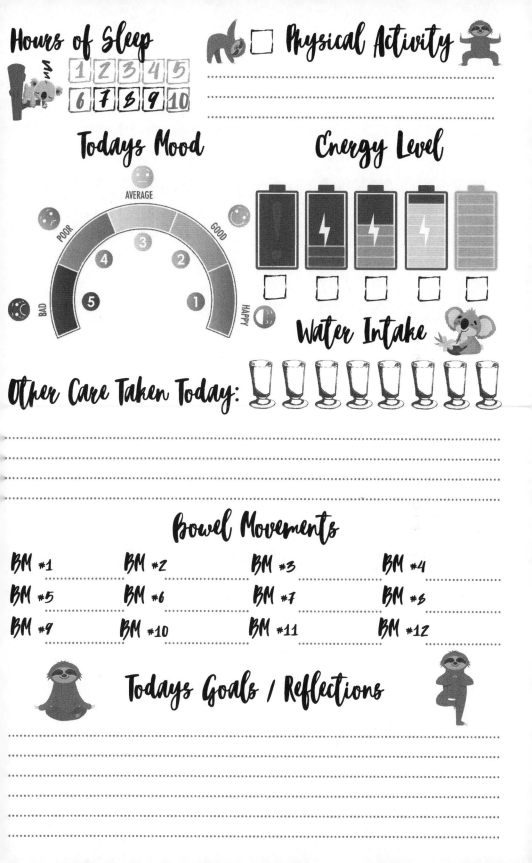

| 1 | 2 | 3 | 4 | 5 |
| 6 | 7 | 8 | 9 | 10 |

Physical Activity

....
....
....

Todays Mood

AVERAGE

POOR

GOOD

3

4   2

BAD

5   1

HAPPY

Energy Level

☐   ☐   ☐   ☐   ☐

Water Intake

Other Care Taken Today:

....
....
....
....

Bowel Movements

BM #1   BM #2   BM #3   BM #4

BM #5   BM #6   BM #7   BM #8

BM #9   BM #10   BM #11   BM #12

Todays Goals / Reflections

....
....
....
....
....

DATE _____ WEIGHT _____

BREAKFAST

....
....
....

TIME _____

PAIN LEVEL ① ② ③ ④ ⑤ ⑥ ⑦ ⑧ ⑨ ⑩

SYMPTOMS

☐ BLOODY STOOLS ☐ DIARRHEA
☐ ABDOMINAL PAIN ☐ FATIGUE
☐ REDUCED APPETITE ☐ WEIGHT LOSS
☐ .... ☐ ....

LUNCH

....
....
....

TIME _____

PAIN LEVEL ① ② ③ ④ ⑤ ⑥ ⑦ ⑧ ⑨ ⑩

SYMPTOMS

☐ BLOODY STOOLS ☐ DIARRHEA
☐ ABDOMINAL PAIN ☐ FATIGUE
☐ REDUCED APPETITE ☐ WEIGHT LOSS
☐ .... ☐ ....

DINNER

....
....
....

TIME _____

PAIN LEVEL ① ② ③ ④ ⑤ ⑥ ⑦ ⑧ ⑨ ⑩

SYMPTOMS

☐ BLOODY STOOLS ☐ DIARRHEA
☐ ABDOMINAL PAIN ☐ FATIGUE
☐ REDUCED APPETITE ☐ WEIGHT LOSS
☐ .... ☐ ....

SNACKS

....
....
....

TIME _____

PAIN LEVEL ① ② ③ ④ ⑤ ⑥ ⑦ ⑧ ⑨ ⑩

SYMPTOMS

☐ BLOODY STOOLS ☐ DIARRHEA
☐ ABDOMINAL PAIN ☐ FATIGUE
☐ REDUCED APPETITE ☐ WEIGHT LOSS
☐ .... ☐ ....

SNACKS

....
....
....

TIME _____

PAIN LEVEL ① ② ③ ④ ⑤ ⑥ ⑦ ⑧ ⑨ ⑩

SYMPTOMS

☐ BLOODY STOOLS ☐ DIARRHEA
☐ ABDOMINAL PAIN ☐ FATIGUE
☐ REDUCED APPETITE ☐ WEIGHT LOSS
☐ .... ☐ ....

MEDICATIONS & SUPPLEMENTS

....
....
....
....
....
....
....
....
....
....

EXTRA NOTES

....
....
....
....
....
....
....
....
....
....

Hours of Sleep

| 1 | 2 | 3 | 4 | 5 |
| 6 | 7 | 8 | 9 | 10 |

Physical Activity

....
....
....

Todays Mood

AVERAGE
POOR
GOOD
BAD
HAPPY

3
4
2
5
1

Energy Level

☐ ☐ ☐ ☐ ☐

Water Intake

Other Care Taken Today:

....
....
....
....

Bowel Movements

BM #1   BM #2   BM #3   BM #4

BM #5   BM #6   BM #7   BM #8

BM #9   BM #10   BM #11   BM #12

Todays Goals / Reflections

....
....
....
....
....
....

DATE _____ WEIGHT _____

BREAKFAST

....
....
....

TIME _____

PAIN LEVEL (1)(2)(3)(4)(5)(6)(7)(8)(9)(10)

SYMPTOMS

☐ BLOODY STOOLS   ☐ DIARRHEA
☐ ABDOMINAL PAIN   ☐ FATIGUE
☐ REDUCED APPETITE   ☐ WEIGHT LOSS
☐ ....   ☐ ....

LUNCH

....
....
....

TIME _____

PAIN LEVEL (1)(2)(3)(4)(5)(6)(7)(8)(9)(10)

SYMPTOMS

☐ BLOODY STOOLS   ☐ DIARRHEA
☐ ABDOMINAL PAIN   ☐ FATIGUE
☐ REDUCED APPETITE   ☐ WEIGHT LOSS
☐ ....   ☐ ....

DINNER

....
....
....

TIME _____

PAIN LEVEL (1)(2)(3)(4)(5)(6)(7)(8)(9)(10)

SYMPTOMS

☐ BLOODY STOOLS   ☐ DIARRHEA
☐ ABDOMINAL PAIN   ☐ FATIGUE
☐ REDUCED APPETITE   ☐ WEIGHT LOSS
☐ ....   ☐ ....

SNACKS

....
....
....

TIME _____

PAIN LEVEL (1)(2)(3)(4)(5)(6)(7)(8)(9)(10)

SYMPTOMS

☐ BLOODY STOOLS   ☐ DIARRHEA
☐ ABDOMINAL PAIN   ☐ FATIGUE
☐ REDUCED APPETITE   ☐ WEIGHT LOSS
☐ ....   ☐ ....

SNACKS

....
....
....

TIME _____

PAIN LEVEL (1)(2)(3)(4)(5)(6)(7)(8)(9)(10)

SYMPTOMS

☐ BLOODY STOOLS   ☐ DIARRHEA
☐ ABDOMINAL PAIN   ☐ FATIGUE
☐ REDUCED APPETITE   ☐ WEIGHT LOSS
☐ ....   ☐ ....

MEDICATIONS & SUPPLEMENTS

....
....
....
....
....
....
....
....

EXTRA NOTES

....
....
....
....
....
....
....
....

Hours of Sleep

1	2	3	4	5
6	7	8	9	10

Physical Activity

☐

....
....
....

Todays Mood

POOR
AVERAGE
GOOD
BAD
HAPPY

3
4
2
5
1

Energy Level

☐ ☐ ☐ ☐ ☐

Water Intake

Other Care Taken Today:

....
....
....
....

Bowel Movements

BM #1	BM #2	BM #3	BM #4
BM #5	BM #6	BM #7	BM #8
BM #9	BM #10	BM #11	BM #12

Todays Goals / Reflections

....
....
....
....
....
....

DATE _____   WEIGHT _____

BREAKFAST

....
....
....
....

TIME _____

PAIN LEVEL ① ② ③ ④ ⑤ ⑥ ⑦ ⑧ ⑨ ⑩

SYMPTOMS

☐ BLOODY STOOLS   ☐ DIARRHEA
☐ ABDOMINAL PAIN   ☐ FATIGUE
☐ REDUCED APPETITE   ☐ WEIGHT LOSS
☐ ....   ☐ ....

LUNCH

....
....
....
....

TIME _____

PAIN LEVEL ① ② ③ ④ ⑤ ⑥ ⑦ ⑧ ⑨ ⑩

SYMPTOMS

☐ BLOODY STOOLS   ☐ DIARRHEA
☐ ABDOMINAL PAIN   ☐ FATIGUE
☐ REDUCED APPETITE   ☐ WEIGHT LOSS
☐ ....   ☐ ....

DINNER

....
....
....
....

TIME _____

PAIN LEVEL ① ② ③ ④ ⑤ ⑥ ⑦ ⑧ ⑨ ⑩

SYMPTOMS

☐ BLOODY STOOLS   ☐ DIARRHEA
☐ ABDOMINAL PAIN   ☐ FATIGUE
☐ REDUCED APPETITE   ☐ WEIGHT LOSS
☐ ....   ☐ ....

SNACKS

....
....
....
....

TIME _____

PAIN LEVEL ① ② ③ ④ ⑤ ⑥ ⑦ ⑧ ⑨ ⑩

SYMPTOMS

☐ BLOODY STOOLS   ☐ DIARRHEA
☐ ABDOMINAL PAIN   ☐ FATIGUE
☐ REDUCED APPETITE   ☐ WEIGHT LOSS
☐ ....   ☐ ....

SNACKS

....
....
....
....

TIME _____

PAIN LEVEL ① ② ③ ④ ⑤ ⑥ ⑦ ⑧ ⑨ ⑩

SYMPTOMS

☐ BLOODY STOOLS   ☐ DIARRHEA
☐ ABDOMINAL PAIN   ☐ FATIGUE
☐ REDUCED APPETITE   ☐ WEIGHT LOSS
☐ ....   ☐ ....

MEDICATIONS & SUPPLEMENTS

....
....
....
....
....
....
....
....
....
....
....

EXTRA NOTES

....
....
....
....
....
....
....
....
....
....
....

Hours of Sleep

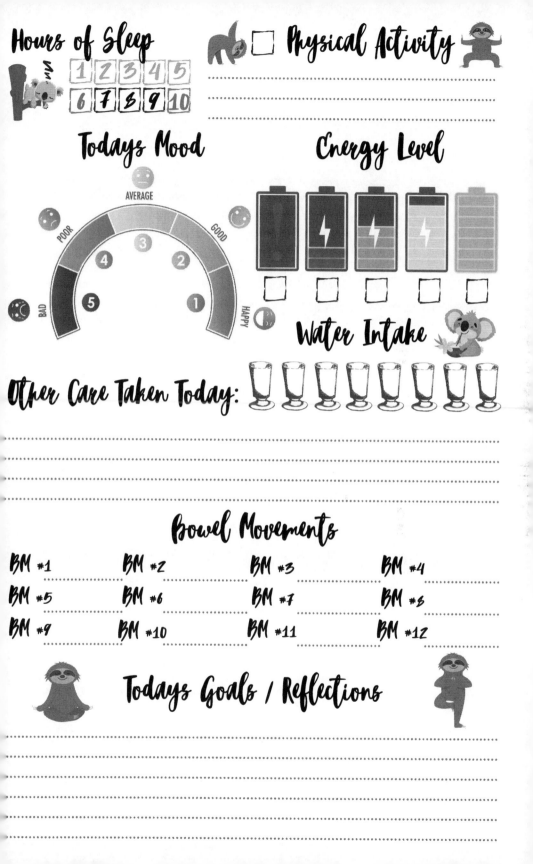

| 1 | 2 | 3 | 4 | 5 |
| 6 | 7 | 8 | 9 | 10 |

Physical Activity ☐

....
....
....

Todays Mood

AVERAGE

POOR

GOOD

4

3

2

5

1

BAD

HAPPY

Energy Level

☐ ☐ ☐ ☐ ☐

Water Intake

Other Care Taken Today:

....
....
....
....

Bowel Movements

BM #1 .... BM #2 .... BM #3 .... BM #4 ....

BM #5 .... BM #6 .... BM #7 .... BM #8 ....

BM #9 .... BM #10 .... BM #11 .... BM #12 ....

Todays Goals / Reflections

....
....
....
....
....
....

DATE ▨▨▨▨▨▨▨▨▨▨▨▨▨▨ WEIGHT ▨▨▨▨▨▨▨▨▨▨▨▨

BREAKFAST

....
....
....
....

TIME ▨▨▨▨▨▨▨▨▨▨▨▨▨▨▨▨▨▨▨▨

PAIN LEVEL ① ② ③ ④ ⑤ ⑥ ⑦ ⑧ ⑨ ⑩

SYMPTOMS

☐ BLOODY STOOLS   ☐ DIARRHEA

☐ ABDOMINAL PAIN   ☐ FATIGUE

☐ REDUCED APPETITE   ☐ WEIGHT LOSS

☐ ....   ☐ ....

LUNCH

....
....
....
....

TIME ▨▨▨▨▨▨▨▨▨▨▨▨▨▨▨▨▨▨▨▨

PAIN LEVEL ① ② ③ ④ ⑤ ⑥ ⑦ ⑧ ⑨ ⑩

SYMPTOMS

☐ BLOODY STOOLS   ☐ DIARRHEA

☐ ABDOMINAL PAIN   ☐ FATIGUE

☐ REDUCED APPETITE   ☐ WEIGHT LOSS

☐ ....   ☐ ....

DINNER

....
....
....
....

TIME ▨▨▨▨▨▨▨▨▨▨▨▨▨▨▨▨▨▨▨▨

PAIN LEVEL ① ② ③ ④ ⑤ ⑥ ⑦ ⑧ ⑨ ⑩

SYMPTOMS

☐ BLOODY STOOLS   ☐ DIARRHEA

☐ ABDOMINAL PAIN   ☐ FATIGUE

☐ REDUCED APPETITE   ☐ WEIGHT LOSS

☐ ....   ☐ ....

SNACKS

....
....
....
....

TIME ▨▨▨▨▨▨▨▨▨▨▨▨▨▨▨▨▨▨▨▨

PAIN LEVEL ① ② ③ ④ ⑤ ⑥ ⑦ ⑧ ⑨ ⑩

SYMPTOMS

☐ BLOODY STOOLS   ☐ DIARRHEA

☐ ABDOMINAL PAIN   ☐ FATIGUE

☐ REDUCED APPETITE   ☐ WEIGHT LOSS

☐ ....   ☐ ....

SNACKS

....
....
....
....

TIME ▨▨▨▨▨▨▨▨▨▨▨▨▨▨▨▨▨▨▨▨

PAIN LEVEL ① ② ③ ④ ⑤ ⑥ ⑦ ⑧ ⑨ ⑩

SYMPTOMS

☐ BLOODY STOOLS   ☐ DIARRHEA

☐ ABDOMINAL PAIN   ☐ FATIGUE

☐ REDUCED APPETITE   ☐ WEIGHT LOSS

☐ ....   ☐ ....

MEDICATIONS & SUPPLEMENTS

....
....
....
....
....
....
....
....
....
....

EXTRA NOTES

....
....
....
....
....
....
....
....
....
....

Hours of Sleep

1	2	3	4	5
6	7	8	9	10

Physical Activity ☐

....
....
....

Todays Mood

POOR

AVERAGE

GOOD

BAD

HAPPY

3

4

2

5

1

Energy Level

☐ ☐ ☐ ☐ ☐

Water Intake

Other Care Taken Today:

....
....
....
....

Bowel Movements

BM #1 .... BM #2 .... BM #3 .... BM #4 ....

BM #5 .... BM #6 .... BM #7 .... BM #8 ....

BM #9 .... BM #10 .... BM #11 .... BM #12 ....

Todays Goals / Reflections

....
....
....
....
....
....

DATE ▨▨▨▨▨▨▨▨▨▨▨▨▨▨▨▨▨▨▨▨ **WEIGHT** ▨▨▨▨▨▨▨▨▨▨▨▨▨▨▨▨▨▨▨▨

BREAKFAST

....
....
....
....

TIME ▨▨▨▨▨▨▨▨▨▨▨▨▨▨▨▨▨▨

PAIN LEVEL ① ② ③ ④ ⑤ ⑥ ⑦ ⑧ ⑨ ⑩

SYMPTOMS

☐ BLOODY STOOLS ☐ DIARRHEA

☐ ABDOMINAL PAIN ☐ FATIGUE

☐ REDUCED APPETITE ☐ WEIGHT LOSS

☐ .... ☐ ....

LUNCH

....
....
....
....

TIME ▨▨▨▨▨▨▨▨▨▨▨▨▨▨▨▨▨▨

PAIN LEVEL ① ② ③ ④ ⑤ ⑥ ⑦ ⑧ ⑨ ⑩

SYMPTOMS

☐ BLOODY STOOLS ☐ DIARRHEA

☐ ABDOMINAL PAIN ☐ FATIGUE

☐ REDUCED APPETITE ☐ WEIGHT LOSS

☐ .... ☐ ....

DINNER

....
....
....
....

TIME ▨▨▨▨▨▨▨▨▨▨▨▨▨▨▨▨▨▨

PAIN LEVEL ① ② ③ ④ ⑤ ⑥ ⑦ ⑧ ⑨ ⑩

SYMPTOMS

☐ BLOODY STOOLS ☐ DIARRHEA

☐ ABDOMINAL PAIN ☐ FATIGUE

☐ REDUCED APPETITE ☐ WEIGHT LOSS

☐ .... ☐ ....

SNACKS

....
....
....
....

TIME ▨▨▨▨▨▨▨▨▨▨▨▨▨▨▨▨▨▨

PAIN LEVEL ① ② ③ ④ ⑤ ⑥ ⑦ ⑧ ⑨ ⑩

SYMPTOMS

☐ BLOODY STOOLS ☐ DIARRHEA

☐ ABDOMINAL PAIN ☐ FATIGUE

☐ REDUCED APPETITE ☐ WEIGHT LOSS

☐ .... ☐ ....

SNACKS

....
....
....
....

TIME ▨▨▨▨▨▨▨▨▨▨▨▨▨▨▨▨▨▨

PAIN LEVEL ① ② ③ ④ ⑤ ⑥ ⑦ ⑧ ⑨ ⑩

SYMPTOMS

☐ BLOODY STOOLS ☐ DIARRHEA

☐ ABDOMINAL PAIN ☐ FATIGUE

☐ REDUCED APPETITE ☐ WEIGHT LOSS

☐ .... ☐ ....

MEDICATIONS & SUPPLEMENTS

....
....
....
....
....
....
....
....
....
....

EXTRA NOTES

....
....
....
....
....
....
....
....
....
....

Hours of Sleep

| 1 | 2 | 3 | 4 | 5 |
| 6 | 7 | 8 | 9 | 10 |

Physical Activity

☐

....
....

Todays Mood

AVERAGE

POOR

GOOD

3

4

2

BAD

5

1

HAPPY

Energy Level

☐ ☐ ☐ ☐ ☐

Water Intake

Other Care Taken Today:

....
....
....
....

Bowel Movements

BM #1 .... BM #2 .... BM #3 .... BM #4 ....

BM #5 .... BM #6 .... BM #7 .... BM #8 ....

BM #9 .... BM #10 .... BM #11 .... BM #12 ....

Todays Goals / Reflections

....
....
....
....
....

DATE _____   WEIGHT _____

BREAKFAST

....
....
....
....

TIME _____

PAIN LEVEL　①②③④⑤⑥⑦⑧⑨⑩

SYMPTOMS

☐ BLOODY STOOLS　　☐ DIARRHEA
☐ ABDOMINAL PAIN　　☐ FATIGUE
☐ REDUCED APPETITE　☐ WEIGHT LOSS
☐ ....　☐ ....

LUNCH

....
....
....
....

TIME _____

PAIN LEVEL　①②③④⑤⑥⑦⑧⑨⑩

SYMPTOMS

☐ BLOODY STOOLS　　☐ DIARRHEA
☐ ABDOMINAL PAIN　　☐ FATIGUE
☐ REDUCED APPETITE　☐ WEIGHT LOSS
☐ ....　☐ ....

DINNER

....
....
....
....

TIME _____

PAIN LEVEL　①②③④⑤⑥⑦⑧⑨⑩

SYMPTOMS

☐ BLOODY STOOLS　　☐ DIARRHEA
☐ ABDOMINAL PAIN　　☐ FATIGUE
☐ REDUCED APPETITE　☐ WEIGHT LOSS
☐ ....　☐ ....

SNACKS

....
....
....
....

TIME _____

PAIN LEVEL　①②③④⑤⑥⑦⑧⑨⑩

SYMPTOMS

☐ BLOODY STOOLS　　☐ DIARRHEA
☐ ABDOMINAL PAIN　　☐ FATIGUE
☐ REDUCED APPETITE　☐ WEIGHT LOSS
☐ ....　☐ ....

SNACKS

....
....
....
....

TIME _____

PAIN LEVEL　①②③④⑤⑥⑦⑧⑨⑩

SYMPTOMS

☐ BLOODY STOOLS　　☐ DIARRHEA
☐ ABDOMINAL PAIN　　☐ FATIGUE
☐ REDUCED APPETITE　☐ WEIGHT LOSS
☐ ....　☐ ....

MEDICATIONS & SUPPLEMENTS

....
....
....
....
....
....
....
....
....
....
....

EXTRA NOTES

....
....
....
....
....
....
....
....
....
....
....

Hours of Sleep

| 1 | 2 | 3 | 4 | 5 |
| 6 | 7 | 8 | 9 | 10 |

Physical Activity

....
....
....

Todays Mood

AVERAGE
POOR
GOOD
BAD
HAPPY

3
4 2
5 1

Energy Level

☐ ☐ ☐ ☐ ☐

Water Intake

Other Care Taken Today:

....
....
....
....

Bowel Movements

BM #1	BM #2	BM #3	BM #4
BM #5	BM #6	BM #7	BM #8
BM #9	BM #10	BM #11	BM #12

Todays Goals / Reflections

....
....
....
....
....

DATE ░░░░░░░░░░░░░░░░░░░░   **WEIGHT** ░░░░░░░░░░░░░░░░░

BREAKFAST

....
....
....
....

TIME ░░░░░░░░░░░░░

PAIN LEVEL ① ② ③ ④ ⑤ ⑥ ⑦ ⑧ ⑨ ⑩

SYMPTOMS

☐ BLOODY STOOLS ☐ DIARRHEA

☐ ABDOMINAL PAIN ☐ FATIGUE

☐ REDUCED APPETITE ☐ WEIGHT LOSS

☐ .... ☐ ....

LUNCH

....
....
....
....

TIME ░░░░░░░░░░░░░░░░░░░░░░░

PAIN LEVEL ① ② ③ ④ ⑤ ⑥ ⑦ ⑧ ⑨ ⑩

SYMPTOMS

☐ BLOODY STOOLS ☐ DIARRHEA

☐ ABDOMINAL PAIN ☐ FATIGUE

☐ REDUCED APPETITE ☐ WEIGHT LOSS

☐ .... ☐ ....

DINNER

....
....
....
....

TIME ░░░░░░░░░░░░░░░░░░░░░░░

PAIN LEVEL ① ② ③ ④ ⑤ ⑥ ⑦ ⑧ ⑨ ⑩

SYMPTOMS

☐ BLOODY STOOLS ☐ DIARRHEA

☐ ABDOMINAL PAIN ☐ FATIGUE

☐ REDUCED APPETITE ☐ WEIGHT LOSS

☐ .... ☐ ....

SNACKS

....
....
....
....

TIME ░░░░░░░░░░░░░

PAIN LEVEL ① ② ③ ④ ⑤ ⑥ ⑦ ⑧ ⑨ ⑩

SYMPTOMS

☐ BLOODY STOOLS ☐ DIARRHEA

☐ ABDOMINAL PAIN ☐ FATIGUE

☐ REDUCED APPETITE ☐ WEIGHT LOSS

☐ .... ☐ ....

SNACKS

....
....
....
....

TIME ░░░░░░░░░░░░░░░░░░░░░░░

PAIN LEVEL ① ② ③ ④ ⑤ ⑥ ⑦ ⑧ ⑨ ⑩

SYMPTOMS

☐ BLOODY STOOLS ☐ DIARRHEA

☐ ABDOMINAL PAIN ☐ FATIGUE

☐ REDUCED APPETITE ☐ WEIGHT LOSS

☐ .... ☐ ....

MEDICATIONS & SUPPLEMENTS

....
....
....
....
....
....
....
....
....
....

EXTRA NOTES

....
....
....
....
....
....
....
....
....

Hours of Sleep

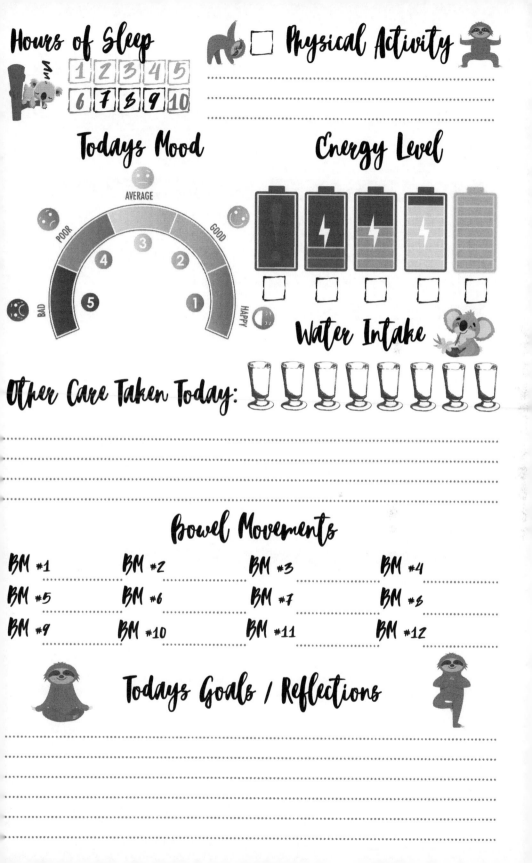

1	2	3	4	5
6	7	8	9	10

Physical Activity

....
....
....
....

Todays Mood

AVERAGE
POOR
GOOD
4   3   2
BAD   5   1   HAPPY

Energy Level

☐   ☐   ☐   ☐   ☐

Water Intake

Other Care Taken Today:

....
....
....
....

Bowel Movements

BM #1	BM #2	BM #3	BM #4
BM #5	BM #6	BM #7	BM #8
BM #9	BM #10	BM #11	BM #12

Todays Goals / Reflections

....
....
....
....
....

DATE _____   **WEIGHT** _____

BREAKFAST

....
....
....
....

TIME _____

PAIN LEVEL ① ② ③ ④ ⑤ ⑥ ⑦ ⑧ ⑨ ⑩

SYMPTOMS

☐ BLOODY STOOLS   ☐ DIARRHEA
☐ ABDOMINAL PAIN   ☐ FATIGUE
☐ REDUCED APPETITE   ☐ WEIGHT LOSS
☐ ....   ☐ ....

LUNCH

....
....
....
....

TIME _____

PAIN LEVEL ① ② ③ ④ ⑤ ⑥ ⑦ ⑧ ⑨ ⑩

SYMPTOMS

☐ BLOODY STOOLS   ☐ DIARRHEA
☐ ABDOMINAL PAIN   ☐ FATIGUE
☐ REDUCED APPETITE   ☐ WEIGHT LOSS
☐ ....   ☐ ....

DINNER

....
....
....
....

TIME _____

PAIN LEVEL ① ② ③ ④ ⑤ ⑥ ⑦ ⑧ ⑨ ⑩

SYMPTOMS

☐ BLOODY STOOLS   ☐ DIARRHEA
☐ ABDOMINAL PAIN   ☐ FATIGUE
☐ REDUCED APPETITE   ☐ WEIGHT LOSS
☐ ....   ☐ ....

SNACKS

....
....
....
....

TIME _____

PAIN LEVEL ① ② ③ ④ ⑤ ⑥ ⑦ ⑧ ⑨ ⑩

SYMPTOMS

☐ BLOODY STOOLS   ☐ DIARRHEA
☐ ABDOMINAL PAIN   ☐ FATIGUE
☐ REDUCED APPETITE   ☐ WEIGHT LOSS
☐ ....   ☐ ....

SNACKS

....
....
....
....

TIME _____

PAIN LEVEL ① ② ③ ④ ⑤ ⑥ ⑦ ⑧ ⑨ ⑩

SYMPTOMS

☐ BLOODY STOOLS   ☐ DIARRHEA
☐ ABDOMINAL PAIN   ☐ FATIGUE
☐ REDUCED APPETITE   ☐ WEIGHT LOSS
☐ ....   ☐ ....

MEDICATIONS & SUPPLEMENTS

....
....
....
....
....
....
....
....
....
....

EXTRA NOTES

....
....
....
....
....
....
....
....
....
....

Hours of Sleep

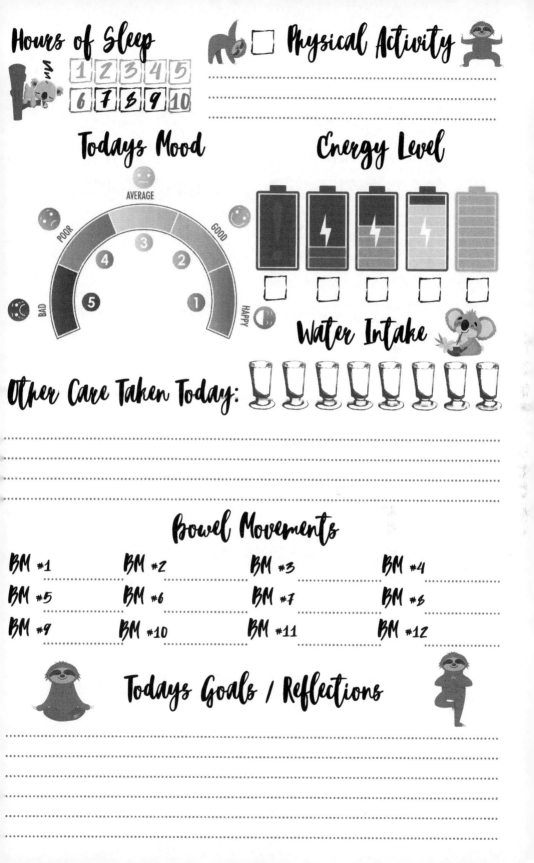

| 1 | 2 | 3 | 4 | 5 |
| 6 | 7 | 8 | 9 | 10 |

☐ Physical Activity

....
....
....

Todays Mood

AVERAGE

POOR

GOOD

BAD

HAPPY

3

4   2

5   1

Energy Level

☐   ☐   ☐   ☐   ☐

Water Intake

Other Care Taken Today:

....
....
....
....

Bowel Movements

BM #1   BM #2   BM #3   BM #4

BM #5   BM #6   BM #7   BM #8

BM #9   BM #10   BM #11   BM #12

Todays Goals / Reflections

....
....
....
....
....

DATE _____   **WEIGHT** _____

BREAKFAST

....
....
....

TIME _____

PAIN LEVEL (1) (2) (3) (4) (5) (6) (7) (8) (9) (10)

SYMPTOMS

☐ BLOODY STOOLS ☐ DIARRHEA
☐ ABDOMINAL PAIN ☐ FATIGUE
☐ REDUCED APPETITE ☐ WEIGHT LOSS
☐ .... ☐ ....

LUNCH

....
....
....

TIME _____

PAIN LEVEL (1) (2) (3) (4) (5) (6) (7) (8) (9) (10)

SYMPTOMS

☐ BLOODY STOOLS ☐ DIARRHEA
☐ ABDOMINAL PAIN ☐ FATIGUE
☐ REDUCED APPETITE ☐ WEIGHT LOSS
☐ .... ☐ ....

DINNER

....
....
....

TIME _____

PAIN LEVEL (1) (2) (3) (4) (5) (6) (7) (8) (9) (10)

SYMPTOMS

☐ BLOODY STOOLS ☐ DIARRHEA
☐ ABDOMINAL PAIN ☐ FATIGUE
☐ REDUCED APPETITE ☐ WEIGHT LOSS
☐ .... ☐ ....

SNACKS

....
....
....

TIME _____

PAIN LEVEL (1) (2) (3) (4) (5) (6) (7) (8) (9) (10)

SYMPTOMS

☐ BLOODY STOOLS ☐ DIARRHEA
☐ ABDOMINAL PAIN ☐ FATIGUE
☐ REDUCED APPETITE ☐ WEIGHT LOSS
☐ .... ☐ ....

SNACKS

....
....
....

TIME _____

PAIN LEVEL (1) (2) (3) (4) (5) (6) (7) (8) (9) (10)

SYMPTOMS

☐ BLOODY STOOLS ☐ DIARRHEA
☐ ABDOMINAL PAIN ☐ FATIGUE
☐ REDUCED APPETITE ☐ WEIGHT LOSS
☐ .... ☐ ....

MEDICATIONS & SUPPLEMENTS

....
....
....
....
....
....
....
....
....

EXTRA NOTES

....
....
....
....
....
....
....
....
....

Hours of Sleep

1	2	3	4	5
6	7	8	9	10

Physical Activity

....
....
....

Todays Mood

AVERAGE
POOR
GOOD
3
4 2
5 1
BAD
HAPPY

Energy Level

☐ ☐ ☐ ☐ ☐

Water Intake

Other Care Taken Today:

....
....
....
....

Bowel Movements

BM #1	BM #2	BM #3	BM #4
BM #5	BM #6	BM #7	BM #8
BM #9	BM #10	BM #11	BM #12

Todays Goals / Reflections

....
....
....
....
....

DATE _____ **WEIGHT** _____

BREAKFAST

....
....
....

TIME _____

PAIN LEVEL ① ② ③ ④ ⑤ ⑥ ⑦ ⑧ ⑨ ⑩

SYMPTOMS

☐ BLOODY STOOLS ☐ DIARRHEA
☐ ABDOMINAL PAIN ☐ FATIGUE
☐ REDUCED APPETITE ☐ WEIGHT LOSS
☐ .... ☐ ....

LUNCH

....
....
....

TIME _____

PAIN LEVEL ① ② ③ ④ ⑤ ⑥ ⑦ ⑧ ⑨ ⑩

SYMPTOMS

☐ BLOODY STOOLS ☐ DIARRHEA
☐ ABDOMINAL PAIN ☐ FATIGUE
☐ REDUCED APPETITE ☐ WEIGHT LOSS
☐ .... ☐ ....

DINNER

....
....
....

TIME _____

PAIN LEVEL ① ② ③ ④ ⑤ ⑥ ⑦ ⑧ ⑨ ⑩

SYMPTOMS

☐ BLOODY STOOLS ☐ DIARRHEA
☐ ABDOMINAL PAIN ☐ FATIGUE
☐ REDUCED APPETITE ☐ WEIGHT LOSS
☐ .... ☐ ....

SNACKS

....
....
....

TIME _____

PAIN LEVEL ① ② ③ ④ ⑤ ⑥ ⑦ ⑧ ⑨ ⑩

SYMPTOMS

☐ BLOODY STOOLS ☐ DIARRHEA
☐ ABDOMINAL PAIN ☐ FATIGUE
☐ REDUCED APPETITE ☐ WEIGHT LOSS
☐ .... ☐ ....

SNACKS

....
....
....

TIME _____

PAIN LEVEL ① ② ③ ④ ⑤ ⑥ ⑦ ⑧ ⑨ ⑩

SYMPTOMS

☐ BLOODY STOOLS ☐ DIARRHEA
☐ ABDOMINAL PAIN ☐ FATIGUE
☐ REDUCED APPETITE ☐ WEIGHT LOSS
☐ .... ☐ ....

MEDICATIONS & SUPPLEMENTS

....
....
....
....
....
....
....
....
....

EXTRA NOTES

....
....
....
....
....
....
....
....
....

Hours of Sleep

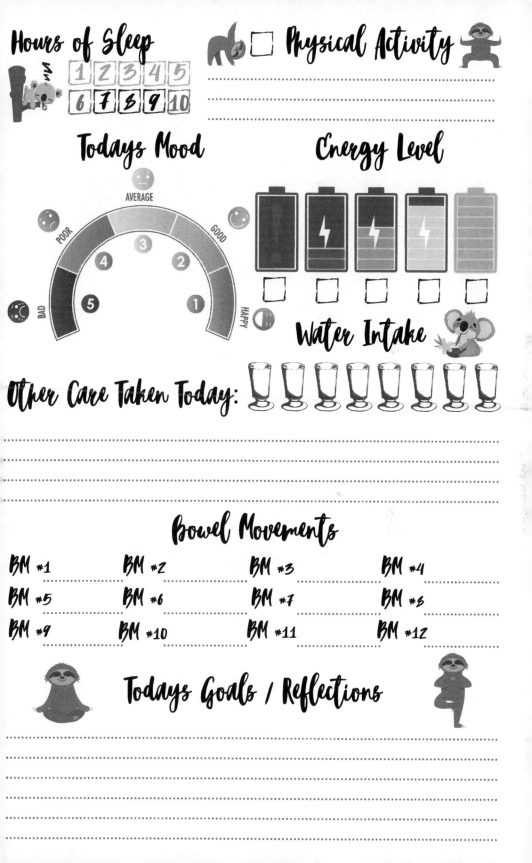

| 1 | 2 | 3 | 4 | 5 |
| 6 | 7 | 8 | 9 | 10 |

Physical Activity

....
....
....

Todays Mood

AVERAGE
POOR
GOOD
3
4 2
BAD 5 1 HAPPY

Energy Level

☐ ☐ ☐ ☐ ☐

Water Intake

Other Care Taken Today:

....
....
....

Bowel Movements

BM #1 .... BM #2 .... BM #3 .... BM #4 ....
BM #5 .... BM #6 .... BM #7 .... BM #8 ....
BM #9 .... BM #10 .... BM #11 .... BM #12 ....

Todays Goals / Reflections

....
....
....
....
....

DATE _____   **WEIGHT** _____

BREAKFAST

....
....
....
....

TIME _____

PAIN LEVEL (1) (2) (3) (4) (5) (6) (7) (8) (9) (10)

SYMPTOMS

- ☐ BLOODY STOOLS
- ☐ ABDOMINAL PAIN
- ☐ REDUCED APPETITE
- ☐ ....
- ☐ DIARRHEA
- ☐ FATIGUE
- ☐ WEIGHT LOSS
- ☐ ....

LUNCH

....
....
....
....

TIME _____

PAIN LEVEL (1) (2) (3) (4) (5) (6) (7) (8) (9) (10)

SYMPTOMS

- ☐ BLOODY STOOLS
- ☐ ABDOMINAL PAIN
- ☐ REDUCED APPETITE
- ☐ ....
- ☐ DIARRHEA
- ☐ FATIGUE
- ☐ WEIGHT LOSS
- ☐ ....

DINNER

....
....
....
....

TIME _____

PAIN LEVEL (1) (2) (3) (4) (5) (6) (7) (8) (9) (10)

SYMPTOMS

- ☐ BLOODY STOOLS
- ☐ ABDOMINAL PAIN
- ☐ REDUCED APPETITE
- ☐ ....
- ☐ DIARRHEA
- ☐ FATIGUE
- ☐ WEIGHT LOSS
- ☐ ....

SNACKS

....
....
....
....

TIME _____

PAIN LEVEL (1) (2) (3) (4) (5) (6) (7) (8) (9) (10)

SYMPTOMS

- ☐ BLOODY STOOLS
- ☐ ABDOMINAL PAIN
- ☐ REDUCED APPETITE
- ☐ ....
- ☐ DIARRHEA
- ☐ FATIGUE
- ☐ WEIGHT LOSS
- ☐ ....

SNACKS

....
....
....
....

TIME _____

PAIN LEVEL (1) (2) (3) (4) (5) (6) (7) (8) (9) (10)

SYMPTOMS

- ☐ BLOODY STOOLS
- ☐ ABDOMINAL PAIN
- ☐ REDUCED APPETITE
- ☐ ....
- ☐ DIARRHEA
- ☐ FATIGUE
- ☐ WEIGHT LOSS
- ☐ ....

MEDICATIONS & SUPPLEMENTS

....
....
....
....
....
....
....
....
....
....

EXTRA NOTES

....
....
....
....
....
....
....
....
....
....

Hours of Sleep

| 1 | 2 | 3 | 4 | 5 |
| 6 | 7 | 8 | 9 | 10 |

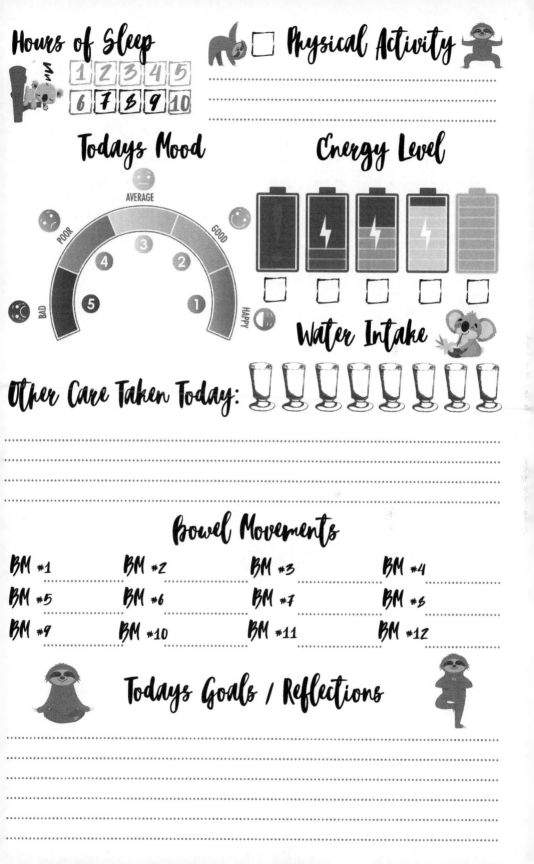

Physical Activity

☐

....
....
....

Todays Mood

AVERAGE
POOR
GOOD
BAD
HAPPY

3
4
2
5
1

Energy Level

☐ ☐ ☐ ☐ ☐

Water Intake

Other Care Taken Today:

....
....
....

Bowel Movements

BM #1	BM #2	BM #3	BM #4
BM #5	BM #6	BM #7	BM #8
BM #9	BM #10	BM #11	BM #12

Todays Goals / Reflections

....
....
....
....
....

DATE _____ **WEIGHT** _____

BREAKFAST

....
....
....

TIME _____

PAIN LEVEL ① ② ③ ④ ⑤ ⑥ ⑦ ⑧ ⑨ ⑩

SYMPTOMS

☐ BLOODY STOOLS ☐ DIARRHEA
☐ ABDOMINAL PAIN ☐ FATIGUE
☐ REDUCED APPETITE ☐ WEIGHT LOSS
☐ .... ☐ ....

LUNCH

....
....
....

TIME _____

PAIN LEVEL ① ② ③ ④ ⑤ ⑥ ⑦ ⑧ ⑨ ⑩

SYMPTOMS

☐ BLOODY STOOLS ☐ DIARRHEA
☐ ABDOMINAL PAIN ☐ FATIGUE
☐ REDUCED APPETITE ☐ WEIGHT LOSS
☐ .... ☐ ....

DINNER

....
....
....

TIME _____

PAIN LEVEL ① ② ③ ④ ⑤ ⑥ ⑦ ⑧ ⑨ ⑩

SYMPTOMS

☐ BLOODY STOOLS ☐ DIARRHEA
☐ ABDOMINAL PAIN ☐ FATIGUE
☐ REDUCED APPETITE ☐ WEIGHT LOSS
☐ .... ☐ ....

SNACKS

....
....
....

TIME _____

PAIN LEVEL ① ② ③ ④ ⑤ ⑥ ⑦ ⑧ ⑨ ⑩

SYMPTOMS

☐ BLOODY STOOLS ☐ DIARRHEA
☐ ABDOMINAL PAIN ☐ FATIGUE
☐ REDUCED APPETITE ☐ WEIGHT LOSS
☐ .... ☐ ....

SNACKS

....
....
....

TIME _____

PAIN LEVEL ① ② ③ ④ ⑤ ⑥ ⑦ ⑧ ⑨ ⑩

SYMPTOMS

☐ BLOODY STOOLS ☐ DIARRHEA
☐ ABDOMINAL PAIN ☐ FATIGUE
☐ REDUCED APPETITE ☐ WEIGHT LOSS
☐ .... ☐ ....

MEDICATIONS & SUPPLEMENTS

....
....
....
....
....
....
....
....
....
....

EXTRA NOTES

....
....
....
....
....
....
....
....
....
....

Hours of Sleep

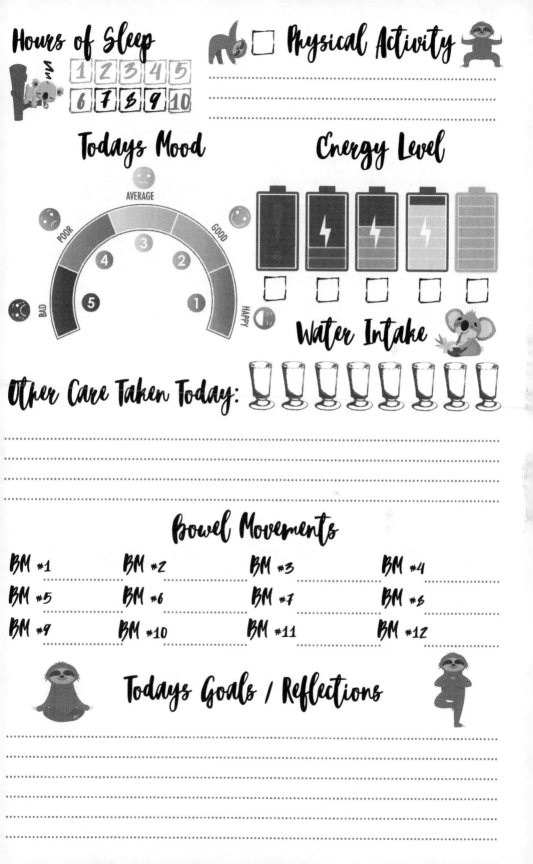

| 1 | 2 | 3 | 4 | 5 |
| 6 | 7 | 8 | 9 | 10 |

☐ Physical Activity

....
....
....

Todays Mood

AVERAGE

POOR

GOOD

3

4

2

BAD

5

1

HAPPY

Energy Level

☐ ☐ ☐ ☐ ☐

Water Intake

Other Care Taken Today:

....
....
....
....

Bowel Movements

BM #1	BM #2	BM #3	BM #4
BM #5	BM #6	BM #7	BM #8
BM #9	BM #10	BM #11	BM #12

Todays Goals / Reflections

....
....
....
....
....

DATE ⬚⬚⬚⬚⬚⬚⬚⬚⬚⬚⬚⬚⬚⬚⬚⬚⬚⬚⬚ **WEIGHT** ⬚⬚⬚⬚⬚⬚⬚⬚⬚⬚⬚⬚⬚⬚

BREAKFAST

....
....
....
....

TIME ⬚⬚⬚⬚⬚⬚⬚⬚⬚⬚⬚⬚⬚⬚⬚⬚⬚

PAIN LEVEL ① ② ③ ④ ⑤ ⑥ ⑦ ⑧ ⑨ ⑩

SYMPTOMS

☐ BLOODY STOOLS ☐ DIARRHEA

☐ ABDOMINAL PAIN ☐ FATIGUE

☐ REDUCED APPETITE ☐ WEIGHT LOSS

☐ .... ☐ ....

LUNCH

....
....
....
....

TIME ⬚⬚⬚⬚⬚⬚⬚⬚⬚⬚⬚⬚⬚⬚⬚⬚⬚

PAIN LEVEL ① ② ③ ④ ⑤ ⑥ ⑦ ⑧ ⑨ ⑩

SYMPTOMS

☐ BLOODY STOOLS ☐ DIARRHEA

☐ ABDOMINAL PAIN ☐ FATIGUE

☐ REDUCED APPETITE ☐ WEIGHT LOSS

☐ .... ☐ ....

DINNER

....
....
....
....

TIME ⬚⬚⬚⬚⬚⬚⬚⬚⬚⬚⬚⬚⬚⬚⬚⬚⬚

PAIN LEVEL ① ② ③ ④ ⑤ ⑥ ⑦ ⑧ ⑨ ⑩

SYMPTOMS

☐ BLOODY STOOLS ☐ DIARRHEA

☐ ABDOMINAL PAIN ☐ FATIGUE

☐ REDUCED APPETITE ☐ WEIGHT LOSS

☐ .... ☐ ....

SNACKS

....
....
....
....

TIME ⬚⬚⬚⬚⬚⬚⬚⬚⬚⬚⬚⬚⬚⬚⬚⬚⬚

PAIN LEVEL ① ② ③ ④ ⑤ ⑥ ⑦ ⑧ ⑨ ⑩

SYMPTOMS

☐ BLOODY STOOLS ☐ DIARRHEA

☐ ABDOMINAL PAIN ☐ FATIGUE

☐ REDUCED APPETITE ☐ WEIGHT LOSS

☐ .... ☐ ....

SNACKS

....
....
....
....

TIME ⬚⬚⬚⬚⬚⬚⬚⬚⬚⬚⬚⬚⬚⬚⬚⬚⬚

PAIN LEVEL ① ② ③ ④ ⑤ ⑥ ⑦ ⑧ ⑨ ⑩

SYMPTOMS

☐ BLOODY STOOLS ☐ DIARRHEA

☐ ABDOMINAL PAIN ☐ FATIGUE

☐ REDUCED APPETITE ☐ WEIGHT LOSS

☐ .... ☐ ....

MEDICATIONS & SUPPLEMENTS

....
....
....
....
....
....
....
....
....
....
....

EXTRA NOTES

....
....
....
....
....
....
....
....
....
....
....

Hours of Sleep

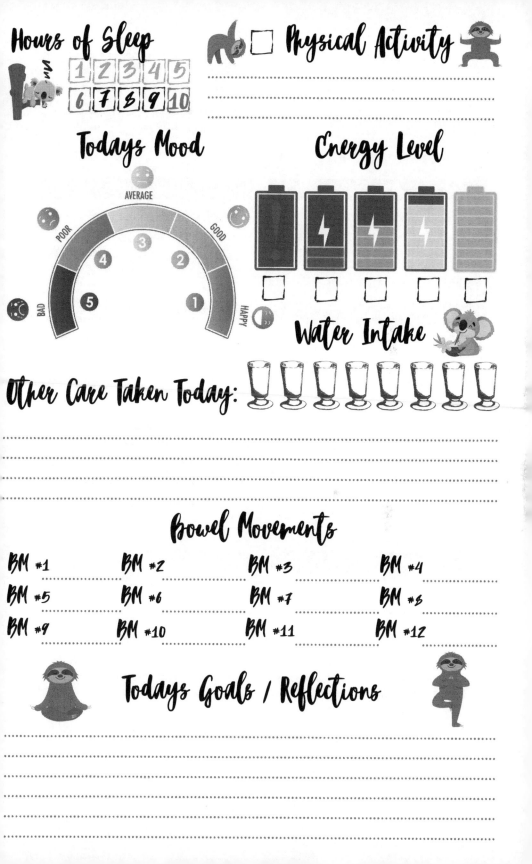

| 1 | 2 | 3 | 4 | 5 |
| 6 | 7 | 8 | 9 | 10 |

☐ Physical Activity

....

....

Todays Mood

AVERAGE

POOR

GOOD

3

4

2

BAD

5

1

HAPPY

Energy Level

☐   ☐   ☐   ☐   ☐

Water Intake

Other Care Taken Today:

....

....

....

Bowel Movements

BM #1   BM #2   BM #3   BM #4

BM #5   BM #6   BM #7   BM #8

BM #9   BM #10   BM #11   BM #12

Todays Goals / Reflections

....

....

....

....

....

....

DATE _____ WEIGHT _____

BREAKFAST

....
....
....
....

TIME _____

PAIN LEVEL ① ② ③ ④ ⑤ ⑥ ⑦ ⑧ ⑨ ⑩

SYMPTOMS

☐ BLOODY STOOLS   ☐ DIARRHEA
☐ ABDOMINAL PAIN   ☐ FATIGUE
☐ REDUCED APPETITE   ☐ WEIGHT LOSS
☐ ....   ☐ ....

LUNCH

....
....
....
....

TIME _____

PAIN LEVEL ① ② ③ ④ ⑤ ⑥ ⑦ ⑧ ⑨ ⑩

SYMPTOMS

☐ BLOODY STOOLS   ☐ DIARRHEA
☐ ABDOMINAL PAIN   ☐ FATIGUE
☐ REDUCED APPETITE   ☐ WEIGHT LOSS
☐ ....   ☐ ....

DINNER

....
....
....
....

TIME _____

PAIN LEVEL ① ② ③ ④ ⑤ ⑥ ⑦ ⑧ ⑨ ⑩

SYMPTOMS

☐ BLOODY STOOLS   ☐ DIARRHEA
☐ ABDOMINAL PAIN   ☐ FATIGUE
☐ REDUCED APPETITE   ☐ WEIGHT LOSS
☐ ....   ☐ ....

SNACKS

....
....
....
....

TIME _____

PAIN LEVEL ① ② ③ ④ ⑤ ⑥ ⑦ ⑧ ⑨ ⑩

SYMPTOMS

☐ BLOODY STOOLS   ☐ DIARRHEA
☐ ABDOMINAL PAIN   ☐ FATIGUE
☐ REDUCED APPETITE   ☐ WEIGHT LOSS
☐ ....   ☐ ....

SNACKS

....
....
....
....

TIME _____

PAIN LEVEL ① ② ③ ④ ⑤ ⑥ ⑦ ⑧ ⑨ ⑩

SYMPTOMS

☐ BLOODY STOOLS   ☐ DIARRHEA
☐ ABDOMINAL PAIN   ☐ FATIGUE
☐ REDUCED APPETITE   ☐ WEIGHT LOSS
☐ ....   ☐ ....

MEDICATIONS & SUPPLEMENTS

....
....
....
....
....
....
....
....
....
....

EXTRA NOTES

....
....
....
....
....
....
....
....
....
....

Hours of Sleep

| 1 | 2 | 3 | 4 | 5 |
| 6 | 7 | 8 | 9 | 10 |

☐ Physical Activity

....
....
....

Todays Mood

AVERAGE

POOR

GOOD

BAD

HAPPY

3

4   2

5   1

Energy Level

☐ ☐ ☐ ☐ ☐

Water Intake

Other Care Taken Today:

....
....
....
....

Bowel Movements

BM #1 .... BM #2 .... BM #3 .... BM #4 ....

BM #5 .... BM #6 .... BM #7 .... BM #8 ....

BM #9 .... BM #10 .... BM #11 .... BM #12 ....

Todays Goals / Reflections

....
....
....
....
....

Printed in Great Britain
by Amazon

35725177R00071